Surviving Mesothelioma and Other Cancers A Patient's Guide

Paul Kraus

Cancer Monthly

Surviving Mesothelioma and Other Cancers:
A Patient's Guide
Paul Kraus

Cancer Monthly, Inc.
14460 New Falls of Neuse Road, Suite 149-243
Raleigh, North Carolina 27614
The Mesothelioma Alliance is a Division of Cancer Monthly, Inc.

Visit our websites:
http//www.cancermonthly.com
http//www.survivingmesothelioma.com
http//www.mycancerplace.com

Library of Congress Control Number: 2005933149

Cataloguing-in-Publication data
Kraus, Paul
Surviving Mesothelioma and Other Cancers:
A Patients Guide
Bibliography.
Includes index.

ISBN 978-0-9772901-1-6

1. Cancer – Patients – Rehabilitation. 2. Cancer – Psychosomatic aspects. 3. Cancer – Social aspects

Cover Photo of Paul Kraus taken in August, 2007 in Newcastle, Australia.

10 9 8 7 6 5 4 3 2

꧁

ACKNOWLEDGMENTS

I would like to thank a number of people who have helped in the writing of this book. Mr. Michael Horwin, M.A., J.D. of Cancer Monthly inspired me with his confidence in this project. I am indebted to him. My wife Sue has not only encouraged and inspired me to put pen to paper but has also been a critical proofreader and a source of much knowledge, especially on the subject of diet and nutritional supplements. Veronica Fenning, senior oncology social worker at the Mater Hospital Newcastle, NSW and Dr. Eckard Roehrich have both been very helpful. Dr. Roehrich's wise counsel and medical skills make him a truly holistic healer. Thanks to all those wonderful people whose lives and works are liberally mentioned in the text, especially Dr. Bernie Siegel and Dr. Andrew Weil, whose writings were like beacons of light during the early days of my illness when the future looked rather bleak.

꧁

DISCLAIMER

ဢ

CONTENTS

FOREWORD

I have been a family physician for over twenty years, with a special interest in holistic medicine. My routine had become somewhat predictable until Paul Kraus came to my office one busy afternoon. I did not suspect that such an unassuming man would lead me to new insights into my understanding of cancer patients.

Despite encouragement given to a number of patients with malignant mesothelioma in my practice over the years, none of them had ever recovered from this cancer, widely regarded as one of the most aggressive and the least treatable of all known cancers. I certainly did not look forward to accepting another case.

Paul had been diagnosed in 1997 with metastases so advanced that the surgeons and cancer specialists had given him no hope of recovery or survival. Paul had been pursuing a holistic treatment approach, simply because orthodox medicine had no more answers for him, except to go home and put his house in order. Imagine my astonishment when I first laid eyes on Paul and found him to be a wiry, strong and rather fit looking man who was in his fourth year of surviving this 'incurable' cancer.

Initially, I just continued the treatments that Paul's previous holistic doctors had carried out and encouraged him to continue his many positive lifestyle changes. His regimen included nutrient therapies, herbal remedies, meditation and exercise, to name just a few. His regimen also included a number of treatment modalities that Paul himself had discovered through the intensive research he had conducted into anti-cancer therapies. Luckily, he was supported in this by his dedicated wife, Sue, who supported Paul in his decision to write about his story and share it with others who might possibly benefit from his experience.

On the surface this book reads like a cookbook, full of practical advice, useful references and guides as how and where to find help after a cancer diagnosis, a most difficult time in anyone's life. Those who read between the lines will find messages that go deeper. Paul's story is not about one or other 'miracle cure' – alternative treatments for cancer frequently fail as do conventional treatments – but how a cancer sufferer can reclaim and enhance his/her life through a holistic approach. Paul addresses social, environmental and spiritual aspects of this illness.

There was more to Paul's story than supplements, treatments and lifestyle changes. As my relationship with Paul unfolded, I discovered that he was willing to probe into the depths of his being and do whatever was necessary to maintain his health, even if that included stress management and painful introspection resulting in personal growth. Paul often mentions the power of faith, hope and love. I would like to add courage to that recipe. I suspect these qualities are the key, while at the same time maintaining a busy and productive lifestyle.

It is impossible to predict the ultimate outcome to what is a most significant health challenge. However, based on his achievements alone, I believe Paul has an important message for us and we should be willing to listen to a person who has defied the odds in such an impressive way. Apart from Paul's many practical and helpful suggestions, there are other powerful messages in his book that I believe will benefit cancer sufferers and health professionals alike.

- Dr. Eckard Roehrich, M.B., B.S., Ph.D.

℘

INTRODUCTION

In June 1997, at the age of 52, I went to my doctor complaining of a protrusion from my navel. Almost instantly he diagnosed an umbilical hernia and referred me to a surgeon to have it repaired. The surgeon assured me that this was a routine minor procedure and there was nothing to worry about. While repairing the hernia, the surgeon noticed a large quantity of fluid leaking from my abdominal cavity. He drained the fluid and conducted an examination with a laparoscope. During that procedure he discovered that I had extensive tumors growing on the peritoneum, the lining of the abdominal wall.

Following the surgery, I was given the grim news that these tumors were not only great in number but that they were also advanced. The surgeon told me quite bluntly that from what he had seen he didn't feel that I had much hope at all. I had advanced cancer, although he could not yet recognize what type of cancer it happened to be.

A definitive diagnosis would have to wait until the results of the pathology were known. This happened almost three weeks following the surgery. The pathologist's report indicated mesothelioma of the peritoneum, the lining of the abdomen.

We quickly learned that pleural and peritoneal mesothelioma were incurable and ultimately fatal, and that my prognosis was less than a year to live. My wife and I were shocked, fearful and feeling very vulnerable in the days, weeks and months following my diagnosis. We sought a number of medical opinions in the quest to know more about what possible treatment options were available. The orthodox therapies of surgery, chemotherapy and radiation therapy were palliative, which meant they were not curative, but were designed to possibly extend survival time.

Unfortunately, these treatments would certainly compromise my quality of life. One oncologist suggested a surgical procedure to de-bulk the tumors. This would necessitate fairly major surgery that included removing the omentum, a large apron that protects the organs of the abdomen. Like the other options, the oncologist warned me that the surgery would not be curative. The problem was that my quality of life was still good and I wanted to keep it that way. Further, we discussed the possibility of surgery with our family doctor who practiced an integrative model of medicine, utilizing conventional and complementary therapies. He was not warm to the suggestion of major surgery. That option was dropped.

My wife and I immediately set about researching as thoroughly as we could every aspect of mesothelioma, as well as cancer in general. I devoted all my energy to convert my ignorance and bewilderment into knowledge that would help me turn this illness around, or at least halt its progress.

In the days following my diagnosis I began a radical lifestyle change that would affect every facet of my life. I commenced a rigorous 'anti-cancer' diet: plenty of fruit and vegetables (predominantly organic), plenty of whole foods – especially grains, nuts, rice and tempeh as well as becoming totally vegetarian. (Tempeh is a food made by the controlled fermentation of cooked soybeans.)

I also began a regime of juicing, starting with four or even five carrot and celery juices each day. I tried to obtain organic carrots whenever possible. The chief rationale for drinking juices was that they are full of nutrients and enzymes that help fight diseases and promote the immune function. Juices also provide instant nutrition as they are readily absorbed. In addition, the carrot juice helped to make my system more alkaline and oxygenate the blood. (An acidic system is not conducive to healing.) Further, the beta carotene is a readily absorbed form of Vitamin A that helps fight cancer.

I avoided refined and processed food, as well as anything fried. I also avoided cane sugar as there is evidence that the glucose molecule is well utilized by cancer cells. The goal of my new nutritional regime was to not only gain premium nourishment but to detoxify the body and thereby give my body the best chance to fight this illness. I also started taking nutritional supplements. This was a regime that I modified quite considerably over time. The mainstay of my treatments was a course of Ukrain (see the chapter on Conventional & Complementary Therapies) and high doses of Vitamin C – both intravenous and oral. This lasted almost two years.

What factors gradually brought acceptance and a slowly growing confidence in my ability to heal? They were numerous. Perhaps the most important of these was my belief that it was not yet my time to go. I was fiercely determined to do everything I could to remain healthy and stay around for a while. My family needed me and I had things to contribute to my fellow human beings. It was simply not my time. The loving support of my wife and two sons was a huge impetus to stay well. I know that love, like hope, has definite physiological side effects and produces endorphins and other hormones that help in the healing process. I read in books such as Dr. Candace Pert's *Molecules of Emotion* of the importance of hope in healing.

I also read widely, not only about cancer and its treatments but, more importantly, inspirational books such as Dr. Bernie Siegel's *Peace Love & Healing* and *Love, Medicine & Miracles* and Dr. Andrew Weil's *Spontaneous Healing.* I learned to meditate and found the benefits of it enormous in helping to balance my life and release me from stress and fear.

With the passing of time I learned, as if by way of a gradual revelation, that healing is a slow process. At times, despite prayer and meditation, I lost perspective on the situation, especially when I presented for a CT scan, which in those early times was almost every three months. My family doctor, whose treatments included hypnotherapy for stress reduction, chided me for being impatient when I complained one day that I was 'still not having any cancer treatment' about four or five months following my diagnosis. He reminded me that the holistic regime I was following was highly therapeutic. Further, the CT scan results and blood test results, although they could have been better, still left me feeling not too bad at all. Despite my distended abdomen from the ascites, or fluid, I had no pain and looked quite well.

Gradually I felt that my condition had stabilized. I listened to what my body was telling me. I exercised daily, as well as visualizing the fluid in my abdomen receding. Intuitively, I knew that my regime was working. All the while I maintained my juicing and diet and did not allow for compromise. I knew that I was battling an illness for which conventional medicine had few answers.

I kept a journal of prose and poetry and found that strategy to be a useful way of expressing my emotions. Whereas my illness had completely dominated my life in those first twelve months I gradually regained my balance and learned to put the illness into perspective. Looking back on those times I find it quite ironic that my cancer diagnosis was, in a strange way, a blessing.

I interpret that event as a sign that God had tapped me on the shoulder and sent me a wake-up call to change the direction of my life. For years, I had been meaning to address those things in my life that were causing me grief, especially my inability to control my stress. I had experienced a fairly major mid-life crisis and left secondary school teaching to buy a business. My attempt at buying a bookstore was, to my deep disappointment, unsuccessful. I compromised by buying a health food store. Little was I to know the long-term consequence of that decision was to help save my life. Going into the health food business gave me a deep interest in natural health and nutrition – knowledge that served me well as I began to fight one of the most dangerous forms of cancer.

Diagnosed with only a few months to live, I am still alive more than twenty years later. The years since my diagnosis have

4

shown that my cancer has been arrested. It no longer grows or spreads. I am not cancer free, but that does not disturb me at all. I have made a choice to live each day in the present moment. That is not to say that I haven't set goals. Rather, it suggests that I have learned to shed the regrets of the past and not to worry about what might happen in the future. Since this watershed in my life I have made a deliberate choice to stay positive.

My spirituality is the foundation of virtually everything else. I now know that there are no coincidences in life. Everything has a purpose and a plan, even when that purpose may be hidden from our eyes. I have learned that life is mysterious and, for the most part, despite the pain and grief that is part of our existence, beautiful. Spirituality is, among other things, the ability to find peace and a sense of purpose in life. It is as much a state of being as a state of mind. I have learned that what Dr. Bernie Siegel calls 'the four faiths' is crucial to recovering from an illness such as cancer: faith in oneself, one's doctor, one's treatment and one's spiritual faith.

Over the years my nutritional supplements: vitamins, minerals, herbs and amino acids have been monitored by my medical herbalist and doctor. My body lets me know when things are not quite right. I spend a great deal of time trying to assist others who find themselves in my predicament. My journey of healing has not been easy, yet it has been a time of great blessing and revelation about living a more fulfilling and joyous life. I thank God for that unexpected watershed day back in mid 1997.

Today, many years after my diagnosis, I remain well. I have far outlived my prognosis and the medical specialist I visited not long ago told me that 'you will be around for a lot longer yet.' My survival has been hard work. The underlying assumption with all that I have done, and continue to do, is a strong belief that our bodies are designed with amazing self-healing capacities. Further, there is much that we can do to maintain wellness. I also believe that we are multi-dimensional beings – mind, body and spirit – and we must nourish each dimension if we are to heal.

It is over twenty years since the healing journey described in this introduction began for me. As I reflect on this time I recall various emotions that came to the fore. They ranged from fear and despair, sadness and disbelief to faith, hope and love. Above all, however, I remember the feeling of determination and empowerment that I felt when my wife and I researched and then began to implement the healing modalities described in these pages. I had nothing to lose as the doctors at that time had nothing to offer. I became convinced that there was much I could do to retain my quality of life and extend my longevity. The prospect of healing this disease was always a consideration.

I knew that getting well again was not some kind of 'quick fix' and so it proved to be. Scans in the six months following diagnosis showed a deterioration in my condition but by twelve months the radiologist would report that the tumors 'appeared unchanged.' I was surprised that my specialist was not as overjoyed as my wife and I at what appeared to be some stabilization of my condition but have since learned that scans can be unreliable and he probably thought the report inaccurate especially as I was defying my prognosis.

An important consideration for anyone on this healing journey is to incorporate products and modalities that you feel are right for you. I was bombarded with so many well-wishers recommending a variety of treatments and while I was happy to research them it was impossible financially or physically to embrace them all. If I thought something offered hope I would use my time of meditation, especially mindful meditation, to make a decision on whether to add it to my regime. As you will read in the book, I believe meditation played an important role in my healing as the mind-body connection is paramount in treating cancer. Interestingly, during the last twenty years the mind-body connection has been validated by many scientific studies. The wonderful aspect about meditation is that as a healing modality it is totally free and therefore available to anyone wishing to use it.

Some years ago I was approached by the wife of a former colleague and she informed me that her husband had been diagnosed with pleural mesothelioma. She told me that

6

financially they were unable to do much in the way of complementary therapies and asked me what I would recommend. I suggested high dose intravenous Vitamin C and also suggested she research the results achieved by a particular integrative clinic. Two years later she phoned to say that her husband had just had a scan and there was no sign of mesothelioma in his lungs. She had taken up my suggestion and he had had no conventional treatment. I share this story, not because Vitamin C is a cure for cancer nor because I am against conventional therapies (I am not), but because it is an example of why it is important to speak to various doctors and clinics to learn about all your options.

In the last twenty years, many people have approached me about what I was doing to survive my mesothelioma. Sadly, some of these individuals were unwilling or unable to consider the complementary path, but as I look back now I am thankful that I was able to maintain the demanding discipline required to stop the disease progressing. My strict lifestyle changes ensured that I stayed alive to see my two sons married and eventually to enjoy my grandchildren. Furthermore, I have been able to pursue a second career in writing and have written a number of books in the past few years and have thoroughly enjoyed my life, despite suffering from two other forms of cancer that were treatable.

I also believe that there is not one healing path that works for everyone. Every patient with mesothelioma needs to find their own path to health. Therefore, the aim of this book is to encourage you to think 'outside the box,' learn how to optimize *your* self-healing capacities and, hopefully, confound the statistics. It describes what worked for me in overcoming my 'terminal' diagnosis and presents my road map to recovery. It is certainly not intended to be a detailed reference book on every type of cancer treatment available (however, there are useful references in the Bibliography) and it in no way purports to provide medical information. Rather, it is written in the framework of addressing the person, not just the illness. It also provides information that in all likelihood your doctor does not have time to give you. Foremost, this book is designed to help you understand that because cancer is life threatening, you need to take it very seriously and 'do whatever it takes' in your fight against it. It also aims to give you the precious commodities of empowerment and hope.

Paul Kraus
Newcastle, 2017

೫ 1 ೞ

A DIAGNOSIS,
NOT A DEATH SENTENCE

THE INITIAL DIAGNOSIS

CANCER, PROBABLY MORE THAN ANY OTHER ILLNESS, STILL CARRIES DEEPLY NEGATIVE SOCIAL BELIEFS. To most people, the word 'cancer' itself induces thoughts of a terminal illness that brings with it the inevitability of pain, suffering and diminished quality and quantity of life. It is a word that is associated with much fear and ignorance. This bias in our thinking suggests that when someone we know is touched by this illness, especially when that 'someone' is in our immediate family, we can easily lose hope. We forget that people have recovered, and do recover, from cancer – even from rare or reasonably advanced forms of cancer that have metastasized (spread from the primary site). We forget that there are many valuable self-help techniques that can bolster whatever medical treatment we may be having. The shock of bad news can blind us to this comforting reality.

In late June 1997, I was quite unexpectedly diagnosed with mesothelioma, the cancer associated with asbestos exposure. It transpired that during the 1960's, when I had a summer job working for a chemical company, that I had indeed been exposed to asbestos. My case was described as peritoneal mesothelioma, as the tumors had disseminated, or seeded, along the peritoneal or abdominal wall. The medical outlook was grim, not only in terms of the prognosis ('a few months – a year at best') but also in terms of the lack of treatments the doctors were able to offer. The surgery my oncologist suggested was intended to prolong my life, not as a curative procedure. Chemotherapy was not an option as I was told that the high dosage would make me very sick and be worse than the illness itself.

The initial shock was followed by confusion and desperation, feelings not helped by a health care system I came to find bewildering and impersonal. The patient and their family are in a highly vulnerable state and often do not know who or what to believe. We tend to listen to anyone who may be in a position to offer hope. Often we go in search of a second, and sometimes a third, medical opinion to confirm the initial diagnosis, particularly if the prognosis is poor. If the medical news remains gloomy we look to alternative therapies for answers.

Immediately after my diagnosis, I began my quest for more knowledge. I went to the bookshop and library and scoured the Health section for useful publications. I surfed the Internet and downloaded every piece of promising information. I listened to people who had experience with this illness. All this in the desperate quest of finding hope where hope is at a premium. Meanwhile I was stalked by fear and a sense of desperation. Fear that the doctor's prognosis was accurate and that my time was running out; fear that I was not making any progress in my quest to find answers to my many questions. I feared that the proposed treatment, surgery, had only a limited likelihood of success. I constantly asked myself what else could I do to give myself the best possible chance of surviving and recovering from this illness. My fear and sense of hopelessness was compounded by my lack of knowledge of available cancer treatments and by a complete ignorance of lifestyle considerations that could help me in the face of this illness. However, I soon came to realize that there were things that I could do to help my situation and to give my body the best possible chance to control this illness and to maintain my quality of life.

I decided to reject the palliative treatments being offered (surgery and chemotherapy) and instead almost immediately following my diagnosis started a rigorous regime of self-help.

(The subject of the remaining chapters.) I learned this regime or "protocol" from a variety of sources including my positive and optimistic family physician and an eminent, if somewhat unusual, cancer surgeon in Melbourne, Australia who viewed medicine as a holistic healing art. (His encouragement was a powerful impetus in my motivation to overcome this illness.)

In addition, about five weeks after my diagnosis my wife and I attended a ten-day retreat for people whose lives had been touched by cancer. This event was an early landmark in my healing journey. We practiced the art of meditation, especially visualization. Here was a highly supportive environment that lacked any judgment or criticism. The participants came from widely diverse backgrounds, but this illness called cancer united us. Some of us were very advanced with this illness and the chances of finding a cure were slender. Others were more fortunate. However, all of us learned many positive things, not merely about how to live with cancer but how to live more fully, more lovingly and how to harness the power of positive emotions such as faith, hope, love and laughter. We also discovered the precious commodity of self-empowerment – taking control of our illness and, indeed, our lives. We learned what it means to have a positive attitude, to accept the diagnosis but to reject the prognosis and not to allow negative thoughts to filter into our belief system. It was at that retreat so soon following my diagnosis that I learned about the blockages to healing, especially guilt, resentment and the lack of forgiveness in one's life. Those ten days were truly self-empowering and gave all of us hope and determination in abundance, as well as the skills to optimize our chances of recovery.

At the first year anniversary after my diagnosis, at the end of June 1998, I greatly rejoiced in the fact that I was alive and well. I wrote a note to the doctor who had given me a matter of months to live to inform him that I was doing fine. I received no response. Although my lifestyle, with its demands on my time and daily routine, precluded me going out into full-time employment, I was able to work as a freelance writer and editor from home. That allowed me the flexibility to maintain my

11

juicing regime, to attend the sessions of intravenous treatment and to give my body the rest it needed. Fatigue was (and remains) a problem, although it is not too debilitating.

Twenty years after I was given "a few months - a year at best" to live, I am still here. My case is perhaps unique, but I would contend that such is every case of cancer.

EVERY CASE IS UNIQUE

Every case of cancer is unique. Many people suffer from the same type of cancer, but there is always a unique set of social and medical variables present with each patient. Some may have had symptoms for only a short while; others may have experienced symptoms for much longer; and still others may not have had any symptoms at all.

No set pattern exists in the events leading up to a cancer diagnosis. Research into the psychosocial factors relating to cancer has indicated that people who have faced some kind of trauma in their lives in the eighteen months or so before a diagnosis are more susceptible to developing cancer. Irrespective of the circumstances surrounding a diagnosis, the actual diagnosis itself is always traumatic. The level of the trauma depends on how the diagnosis is presented to a patient. Some doctors are able to give bad news in such a way that a person does not succumb to despair, while others are too blunt and perhaps a little insensitive about the information they give to the patient and their family. The diagnosis is usually overwhelming, and many patients do not hear anything further that is said during the consultation. A follow-up appointment is always advisable.

The doctor giving the bad news may fail to mention that there are reasons for hope. The news of the diagnosis is usually given as a set of facts relating to what the surgeon or the pathologist found. The subsequent prognosis is based on a combination of clinical and statistical evidence. Few doctors tell the patient that each case is unique and there is a degree of unpredictability in the way the illness will develop. In the tense situation of the consultation at the time of the diagnosis, it is easy to forget that people have recovered from most types of cancer. Some people defy the statistics, defy the odds and make remarkable recoveries. With the accompanying trauma of a cancer diagnosis it is easy to forget that there are self-help techniques that can improve your quality of life and optimize your chances of becoming a long-term survivor. It is only natural that the shock of bad news blinds you to such inspiring truths.

Scientific studies reported in medical journals worldwide attest to the fact that those who take an active role in their illness and adopt self-help techniques improve their chances of recovery. The most important advice following your diagnosis is not to despair and lose hope by believing that the doctor's words represent the whole truth. Nor should you believe that you must begin your treatment immediately. You need time to accept the diagnosis, to come to terms with it and to resolve not to accept the prognosis, especially if it happens to be poor. Again, remember that statistics are only statistics. They are merely figures roughly indicating probabilities – *not certainties.*

Responses to a cancer diagnosis vary widely. Many people experience a reaction not unlike grieving, with various phases including denial – 'It couldn't be me...they've got it wrong,' bargaining, depression and eventually acceptance. As with grieving, people work through these stages at their own pace. Some do not have such a reaction at all. My own cancer diagnosis was one such case. For a number of years prior to it I had lived a very stressful life, a life that lacked balance and inner harmony. While the shock of being diagnosed was profound and shattering (especially because of its accompanying poor prognosis), I recognized that this illness was probably linked to the lack of balance in my life over the past few years.

It would be dishonest of me not to admit to frequent bouts of fear in those early days, weeks and even months after the diagnosis. The fear stemmed from being so suddenly and abruptly confronted by my mortality when I was still relatively young – well at least middle-aged! It was not so much the thought of death that made me afraid; it was the fear of dying. Twenty years earlier I had witnessed the prolonged and painful death of my father from prostate cancer. I feared having to endure his suffering.

Even though I did have moments of denial, or rather disbelief, in those early days, I was fortunate enough to be able to accept the diagnosis quickly. Only by accepting my situation was I able to confront certain fundamental choices. The foremost of these was making up my mind to do everything in my power to get well again. I wanted to live. I had strong reasons for wanting to live, for hoping to enjoy life still, to enjoy my family and of being of some use to my fellow human beings. I had no trouble resolving that there was much to look forward to in life.

Preceding the acceptance phase of my diagnosis was a deep hope in my recovery – that indeed, the doctor's diagnosis did not necessarily mean that I was at the end of the road. In numerous ways I learned that hope is therapeutic to the human spirit and that anything which is therapeutic to the spirit is also therapeutic to the body. I quickly learned that there is always something to hope for in the face of a difficult illness. I also experienced the healing power of faith, of love and of laughter. These important healing emotions are the subject of the next chapter about the principles of healing. They are also the subject of my book, *Faith, Hope, Love and Laughter: How They Heal* (see Bibliography). It is important to realize the link between our thoughts and our physical wellbeing. I knew that I couldn't afford to wallow in self-pity or despair or to dwell on the negative. Negativity would mean succumbing to my illness. It would also lead to a dramatically reduced quality of life and probably quantity of life as well.

QUESTIONS TO ASK YOUR DOCTOR

The trauma of a cancer diagnosis leaves confusion in its wake. Your doctor will usually recommend that you see an oncologist. It is perfectly understandable that following the diagnosis of a life-threatening illness such as cancer you would want to have a second opinion, not only to confirm the diagnosis but also to investigate the most effective form of treatment.

Usually your family physician will oblige and be able to recommend a specialist. Right from the beginning, ask your doctor for a copy of all your test results. You have a right to do this. Keeping a folder with your pathology report, blood tests, scan reports (MRI's, CT's, etc.) and other results is invaluable for showing another doctor the medical history of your illness should you want to have additional medical opinions.

Useful questions to ask your oncologist include:

- What is the exact type of cancer I have and how prevalent is it?

- To what extent has the cancer spread beyond the primary site, if at all?

- Has only one organ been affected or is there further involvement?

- Is there a need for a second pathologist to review the initial findings? (It is often advisable to have pathologists from at least two separate institutions review your "slides" to confirm the pathology diagnosis as mistakes can be made with the initial diagnosis.)

- Is there any need for additional tests? If so, what are you looking for in such tests?

- How can you be absolutely certain that the test results are accurate?

- What are my treatment options? Which ones do you recommend?

- What success rate does the treatment have? Will the treatment be a cure?

- What are the potential short-term and long-term side-effects of the treatment in question?

Remember that you have every right to ask these questions. After all, your aim is to make informed treatment decisions and receive the best treatment available.

UNDERSTAND YOUR TREATMENT OPTIONS

Most mainstream cancer treatment options fall into one of the following categories: *surgery*, *chemotherapy*, or *radiation therapy*.

Surgery is probably the most common form of cancer treatment. In pleural mesothelioma, the most frequent surgeries performed are Extrapleural Pneumonectomy or EPP and Pleurectomy / Decortication or PD. For peritoneal mesothelioma, the most frequent surgery is heated intraperitoneal chemotherapy or HIPEC procedure.

SURGERY FOR PLEURAL MESOTHELIOMA

An Extrapleural Pneumonectomy or EPP is the most invasive surgery for mesothelioma and involves the removal of the diseased lung, part of the pericardium, (the membrane that covers the heart), part of the diaphragm (the muscle that lies between the abdomen and the lungs), and part of the parietal pleura (this is the membrane that lines the chest). An EPP is typically performed only on patients with early stage localized disease that has not metastasized to the lymph nodes or to other tissues and organs. Sometimes heated chemotherapy is introduced during an EPP in order to bathe affected tissues. Although an EPP can impact life expectancy for some patients, there can be significant risks to this procedure. These risks may include: internal bleeding, respiratory failure, infection and blood clots. In addition, some patients undergoing extrapleural pneumonectomy die during or immediately following the

16

procedure. That percentage is, however, lower at medical centers that specialize in this surgery.

Pleurectomy / Decortication (PD) refers to a lung-sparring surgery to remove the mesothelioma cancer by removing part of the covering of the lungs, lining of the chest, and part of the outside surface of the lungs. The goals of the operation are to re-expand the lung and remove the disease process affecting the pleural space so that pulmonary (lung) function and symptoms will improve.

Other, more modest, surgical procedures include Pleurocentesis and Pleurodesis. Pleurocentesis is used to minimize pleural effusion, the build-up of fluid in the pleural space surrounding the lungs. The fluid can make it difficult for a mesothelioma patient to breath. The procedure involves the surgical puncture and drainage of the thoracic cavity and is usually performed in an outpatient setting with a long, thin needle that is inserted into the pleural space. Pleurodesis is a surgical procedure that uses chemicals, talc or drugs to scar the space between the layers of the pleura. First, fluid is drained from the space using a catheter or chest tube. Next, the chemical, talc or drug is put into the space. The scarring stops the build-up of fluid in the pleural cavity. This is sometimes referred to as a "talc procedure."

SURGERY FOR PERITONEAL MESOTHELIOMA

Surgical procedures for peritoneal mesothelioma include paracentesis, Peritonectomy / Cytoreductive Surgery, and HIPEC.

Similar to pleurocentesis, paracentesis is a procedure in which fluid from the abdomen is removed through a needle. It is performed on peritoneal mesothelioma patients to remove pressure from the fluid.

Peritonectomy is the most common surgical procedure for peritoneal mesothelioma and involves the removal or stripping of the affected peritoneum (cancerous part of the lining of the abdominal cavity) from the underlying tissue. Peritonectomy is usually combined with cytoreductive surgery where the goal is to also remove as much of the cancerous growth as possible from multiple sites in the abdomen. The greater omentum is nearly always involved and has to be removed.

Doctors often perform cytoreductive surgery in combination with other mesothelioma treatments such a chemotherapy. For example, in a HIPEC procedure (heated intraperitoneal chemotherapy), surgeons introduce heated chemotherapy directly into the surgical cavity. In the peer reviewed medical literature, HIPEC procedures used in peritoneal mesothelioma management report superior survival statistics when compared to other surgeries.

CHEMOTHERAPY

Chemotherapy is a group of toxic drugs that kill cells (mesothelioma, other cancers, and healthy cells) by damaging their DNA. Chemotherapy is a cytotoxic therapy, meaning it kills cells. Chemo drugs target rapidly growing cancer cells, but they can also affect healthy cells that grow rapidly such as blood cells. The effect of these drugs on both cancer and normal cells often causes side effects.

As of this writing, the only FDA approved chemotherapy for mesothelioma is a combination of Alimta (pemetrexed) and cisplatin. In February 2004, the Food and Drug Administration approved pemetrexed for the treatment of malignant pleural mesothelioma in combination with cisplatin for patients whose disease is either inoperable or who are not otherwise candidates for curative surgery. Patients who take this chemo regimen are often prescribed folic acid and vitamin B12 supplement to help reduce side effects from the chemotherapy. Patients are usually prescribed corticosteroids to reduce the risk of skin rashes as well.

There was one key clinical trial that led to the FDA approval of this regimen for mesothelioma. Two hundred twenty-six pleural mesothelioma patients were randomized to receive pemetrexed and cisplatin, while 222 patients were randomized to receive cisplatin alone. The primary study end point was survival. Median survival times were 12.1 months for the pemetrexed plus cisplatin treatment group and 9.3 months for the cisplatin alone group.

Median time to progression (regrowth of tumor) was longer in the pemetrexed/cisplatin arm of the study, 5.7 months versus 3.9 months. This means that the mesothelioma patients who received both drugs had their tumors return a median of 1.8 months longer versus those who only got one drug.

Like most chemo drugs, pemetrexed kills blood cells so the most common adverse events were neutropenia, fatigue, leukopenia, nausea, dyspnea, and vomiting.

RADIATION THERAPY

Radiation therapy may sometimes be used as part of a "multi-modality" approach. This means that radiation therapy may be added to other treatments such as surgery and chemotherapy. Radiation such as x-rays or gamma rays may be delivered externally via external beam radiation. Radiation can also be delivered internally by placing radioactive substances such as cesium, iridium, and iodine near or into cancerous tissue within the body or administering radionuclides systemically (into the bloodstream).

IMPORTANT QUESTIONS

Important questions to ask your doctor about any of these treatments include:

- What is the efficacy (effectiveness)?

- Is the treatment curative (designed to cure) or palliative (designed to improve symptoms)?

- What side effects can I expect?

19

- How long does the treatment last?'

The above three treatment modalities are the major "conventional," "orthodox" or "mainstream" treatment options. The success rate or "efficacy" of these modalities is often limited in mesothelioma and other advanced, aggressive, and metastatic cancers. Therefore, it is important to always ask about the success rate of the treatment that is being recommended. It is an interesting fact that the efficacy of some of the conventional therapies, especially chemotherapy, has not substantially improved over the past few decades. Therefore, it is critical to be fully aware of what is involved in a course of treatment both in terms of efficacy and toxicity (side-effects).

Although the vast majority of cancer patients are treated by one of these conventional methods, recent studies have revealed that an increasing number of cancer patients are turning to some form of complementary therapy as well. (See for example Richardson, et al., "Complementary/Alternative Medicine Use in a Comprehensive Cancer Center and the Implications for Oncology," *Journal of Clinical Oncology*, July 2000.) Most oncologists discourage their patients from using complementary therapies, claiming that they are scientifically 'unproven' and using them is a waste of money and will not improve the chances of survival or recovery. Many physicians do not realize that when a patient strongly believes that a treatment is working, then that in itself must be considered beneficial, however 'unscientific' it is deemed to be. Nonetheless, as with any profession, there are poorly qualified and unscrupulous natural therapists who are only too willing to prescribe expensive treatments that are of dubious merit. (More on Complementary Therapies in Chapter 4.)

Whether you choose conventional or complementary therapies, the most important aspect of going with a particular treatment is that you believe in it and have full confidence that it will work. Likewise, you need to have a good rapport and full confidence in your doctor, whether he or she happens to be a family physician, holistic practitioner, or orthodox oncologist.

Remember that if your doctor frowns on any complementary treatment you may be having, then do not necessarily be deterred. Most mainstream physicians are untrained in the potential efficacy of these therapies. Definitely cease that treatment, however, if your doctor states that it would interfere with the treatment you have already decided on. Whatever treatment you consent to having, whether orthodox or complementary, find out as much as you can about it. The more you understand about your treatment, the more positive you can be that it will work for you.

THE DOCTOR–PATIENT RELATIONSHIP

Shortly after my diagnosis I made a point of writing down my questions and concerns before the visits to the doctor. I was fortunate to be accompanied by my wife. Two pairs of ears are better than one. It is always advisable to ask your partner to take brief notes of the answers to your questions. If you have a long list of questions ask if it is possible to have extra time with the doctor during your appointment. If you have difficulty communicating with your doctor, express this concern. If the rapport does not improve then be prepared to change physicians. Be absolutely honest at all times, but bear in mind that an oncologist will not have had any training (or at best very little) in diet, nutrition and nutritional therapies. Also, she will probably have a bias against so-called 'unproven' therapies.

In his best-selling book *Peace, Love and Healing*, Bernie Siegel, MD devotes an entire chapter to the doctor–patient relationship. From a cancer patient's perspective, the reason is not hard to see. The patient's faith in his doctor is a vital determinant in his ability to heal. Fundamental to that relationship is that patients want to be seen as people, not as statistics. This may sound too idealistic because of the pressures facing most doctors today, yet its truth is undeniable. A patient presenting with a life-threatening illness such as cancer is not only looking for a treatment that will help to put them on a healing path, they want to be able to relate freely with their doctor and not be afraid to ask questions that are of genuine concern. The doctor who has patients in and out of her room in the shortest possible time is hardly in a position to develop a genuine rapport with you. As one of Dr. Siegel's patients once remarked: 'Surgery visits are okay but I need to know how to live between surgery visits...' Again, maybe this sounds too idealistic, indeed, unrealistic, but even a few words of reassurance, a brief conversation, a smile and a few words of hope can do wonders for a patient, whether or not he or she is suffering from a life threatening illness.

A doctor who is not merely a mechanistic practitioner but also a healer is sensitive to your physical, psychological and spiritual welfare. Lack of communication between you and your doctor impedes the healing process. You have a right to be well informed. Do not feel intimidated.

I was very fortunate in that I had a doctor (my family physician) whose approach to cancer treatment reflected my own beliefs. (Had there been a conventional treatment that stood a good chance of curing my illness, I would have integrated it with other non-conventional therapies.) I had decided to pursue a path of holistic care, using relaxation, meditation, diet, herbs, vitamins, and other supplements and my doctor was able and willing to facilitate this course of treatment.

I had established an excellent rapport with him. This meant that I could freely discuss with him the pros and cons of what I was doing, as well as ask him questions about other treatments that I was considering. While this type of physician may be in the minority, they do exist in every country and can be identified with a little research. The important point is to have a doctor who can facilitate your treatment decisions and care for you as a person not a tumor. If you opt for conventional treatments you deserve a doctor who not only can prescribe chemotherapy, radiation, or surgery, but can also take the time to explain the impact of these treatments and patiently answer your questions. If you decide on holistic care you deserve a practitioner who can explore with you all avenues of healing.

SUPPORT GROUPS

Speaking to others who are undergoing a similar treatment as you can be reassuring. This is one of the benefits of belonging to a cancer support group. Find and join a support group. Sharing your apprehensions and fears is an important way of allaying them. Always remember that hope has positive physiological side effects. The more hope you have, the better you will feel. A positive approach to your illness and to your outlook on life will increase your chances of recovery.

MEDITATION

There are some who would argue that meditation is not a therapy. Yet research on the effects of meditation and deep relaxation on the body strongly suggests that it has powerful therapeutic effects in terms of helping to improve immune function. In the early 1970's Dr. Ainslie Meares, an Australian psychiatrist, pioneered the use of meditation as an adjunctive cancer therapy. He published his findings in the *Medical Journal of Australia,* but his colleagues (especially in the oncology field), remained unconvinced. A few years later, the *Lancet*, one of the world's most respected medical journals, also published Meares' research.

Meares wrote more than twenty books, including a number on the benefits of meditation. His book *The Wealth Within* and *Cancer – Another Way?* offers fascinating and valuable insights into the way our bodies heal. *Cancer: Another Way?* is a highly inspirational book, written in simple short verse. Although it is now out of print, Amazon, libraries and some second-hand bookshops may have copies.

Meares' best-known patient was Ian Gawler, a young veterinary surgeon who developed an aggressive and usually fatal osteogenic sarcoma in 1975. Gawler's cancer spread, despite the amputation of his right leg. By 1976, he was critically ill and close to death. Meares helped Gawler adopt a number of intensive meditation techniques, both passive and active, as well as a range of radical dietary treatments. Gradually, Gawler's condition improved. Within three years he was declared 'free of active neoplastic disease' (cancer). In 1978, Meares documented Gawler's case in the *Medical Journal of Australia*.

Meditation has, at various times, been called a 'silent healer' because it optimizes the body's self-healing potential and mechanisms. At its simplest, it does this by reducing stress levels and lowering the metabolic rate. The main physical benefit of meditation is that it decreases the adrenalin and cortisone output of the endocrine system. Studies have revealed that negative emotions such as fear do, in fact, alter the body's chemistry. Small wonder then that prolonged or acute stress often leads to illness, as occasionally happens after bereavement. The immune response is lowered and the body is susceptible to infection. Meditation complements the benefit of any treatment, conventional or complementary, that you may be having, by profoundly relaxing the body. It is a simple, pleasant and highly efficient way of advancing the healing process. It is practiced quite independently of whatever religious belief you might hold. One doctor in the United States has described meditation as 'breaking our addiction to thought,' stopping our incessantly chattering minds and 'letting go' of our fears and anxieties. It is also the art of anchoring ourselves in the present moment – a very valuable thing to be able to do following a cancer diagnosis. (More on meditation in Chapter 6.)

CHAPTER SUMMARY

- A cancer diagnosis brings with it acute stress. We feel bewildered and desperate. We want answers to our many questions. Fear of rapid progression of the disease and all that it entails is an abiding worry. Will I live with pain? Will my treatment work? Do I really trust my doctor's judgments?

- Self-help techniques exist that can optimize your chances of becoming a long-term cancer survivor. It is vital for your peace of mind to *accept the diagnosis but to reject the prognosis.* The prognosis is based on statistics. There is much you can do to beat the statistics. Above all, think positively and avoid projecting your fears into the future. Live in the present.

- Hope has physiological side effects. Never give up. People have recovered from very difficult situations and beaten the odds. If remarkable recoveries have occurred with others, they can occur with you. Your attitude is of paramount importance! Read stories of inspiring people who have beaten the odds.

- Do not be afraid to ask your doctor the questions that are worrying you. Develop a good rapport with your healthcare provider. It is vital to have a firm faith in your doctor and in your treatment. If these are missing, then find another doctor. Understand your treatment options.

- You can enhance the beneficial effects of whatever treatment you are having by making life-affirming choices such as meditation, an anti-cancer diet and by taking nutritional supplements. Be aware that you are a spiritual being.

- Beware of those who, with the best of intentions, tell you to try this or that 'cancer cure.' Thoroughly check the credentials of any practitioner who offers you treatment. However, do begin any self-help technique that will aid in your overall healing. (Remember that positive thinking and meditation are free.)

ഇ 2 രൂ

THE EMOTIONAL AND SPIRITUAL PRINCIPLES OF HEALING

IT SEEMS THAT ONLY WHEN A LIFE-THREATENING ILLNESS SUCH AS CANCER TOUCHES OUR LIVES DO WE STOP TO THINK HOW OFTEN WE TAKE HEALTH FOR GRANTED. We rarely, if at all, think about actively promoting 'wellness.' What, then, is wellness? It is far more than an absence of illness. Rather, it is part of enjoying a harmonious balance between body, mind and emotions. As we get older and life inevitably throws a plentiful supply of challenges our way and we encounter the rough and tumble of life, with its joys, pains and sorrows, 'wellness' seems more and more elusive. Provided we do not succumb to illness, we rarely think about promoting health, even when we realize that our life lacks balance and harmony. Sometimes, when we live in a state of stress, or what some health professionals call 'dis-ease' for a lengthy period of time, our bodies rebel and we develop a chronic illness such as cancer.

Carcinogenic substances such as asbestos, coal tar from cigarettes, certain dyes and other chemicals have been linked to the incidence of various types of cancers. Yet the question remains as to why only some of those who are exposed to such toxic substances develop the disease while others do not. Are they in some way genetically predisposed? Various theories over many years have been put forward regarding this question. It seems likely that genetic factors do play a part – but only a part. Psychological and medical studies worldwide have also indicated a link between stress, personality type, and cancer. The link is all the more marked when stress has accumulated in a person's life and he has succumbed to a sense of hopelessness. It is as if the body's immune function becomes impaired and loses its ability to ward off illness. Anxiety, stress and a sense of hopelessness exhaust the adrenal glands, upset the body's hormonal balance and thus impair the immune system. Simply stated, this is the basis of the physiology of stress. The surprising thing is that the medical profession seems slow, even reluctant, to acknowledge this link.

PERSONALITY, STRESS AND CANCER

We cannot begin a journey of healing unless we realize that there is a connection between our 'inner environment' – our state of mind – and our physical well-being.

In the early 1970's Dr. Lawrence Le Shan, an experimental psychologist in the United States, published a book on his research into the background of cancer patients called *You Can Fight for Your Life: Emotional Factors in the Causation of Cancer*. Included in Le Shan's findings is what he termed a typical personality profile of cancer patients. He found that they tended to be introverted people who had undergone stress in their childhood and youth. They tended to be people who had difficulty in expressing their feelings to others, especially to those close to them. They frequently experienced unresolved emotional conflicts and had residual anger, frustration and hurt. His findings also suggested that they had difficulty in coping with life's circumstances and felt that they were indeed the victims of circumstance. Not infrequently a sense of hopelessness had been a part of their life, especially eighteen months or so before the diagnosis. Many research studies have been done since Le Shan's findings were first published. The majority of these studies confirm the typical psychological profile of cancer patients.

If we accept that there is frequently a connection between personality and cancer we can recognize a cancer diagnosis as a wake-up call to change our lifestyles, to change our belief systems, to begin learning how to affirm the positive aspects of our lives and to delete the negatives. We need to learn to let go of fear and other negative emotions that adversely affect our health. This may not be easy, but it is vital if we are to improve our quality of life and be one of those people who survives against the odds and recovers from their illness.

The day after I was unexpectedly diagnosed with cancer I went to see my family physician. Not surprisingly, I was in a state of shock and emotionally at rock bottom, having just been told by my surgeon that there was not much that medicine could do for me. In contrast, my family physician's calm words of reassurance and hope were like a healing balm. At the end of the consultation he reached for his script pad and began writing a list. I assumed he was prescribing medications. When he had finished writing he looked at me and explained what he had just written.

His list began with the name of a book that I should begin reading as soon as possible. It was *Getting Well Again*, by Carl and Stephanie Simonton. The list included such things as getting a pet (which I already owned), squeezing a rubber stress ball while listening to soft music daily, exercising daily and watching a funny movie and having a good laugh. I have to admit to feeling a little indignant at his list of recommendations. I was desperately looking for practical advice, for actual treatment options, not for some airy-fairy 'feel-good' strategies. He said quite unambiguously and with the utmost seriousness that these things were very important if I hoped to begin healing. Indeed, they were part of my treatment options!

Within the following week, he began a series of sessions with me in which he taught me the basics of 'letting go' through the gentle healing art of meditation. I had to admit that after these sessions I did feel considerably better and more relaxed. My doctor helped me to discover aspects of a healing lifestyle previously foreign to me.

FAITH – THE FORGOTTEN FACTOR IN HEALING

Before looking at the meaning and importance of having a positive mindset when confronted by cancer (and how to translate that mindset into action), I want to mention briefly the role of faith in helping us to let go of the ever-present fear that comes with a cancer diagnosis. While doctors may often talk about having a positive attitude and about thinking positively they rarely mention the word 'faith.' Yet, ironically, there is plenty of research data from clinical psychology and psychiatry journals to show that faith is not a sugar-coated placebo but rather is a scientifically proven aid to healing. It is surprising to think that faith is a scientifically validated tool to improve medical outcomes but evidence exists to show that this is the case. For example, evidence about the 'faith factor' in healing is cited in *Healing Words, The Power of Prayer & The Practice of Medicine* by Larry Dossey, MD (Harper Collins, New York, 1993).

In this context I define faith as a spiritual commitment, a relationship and communication with your concept of God; a belief in a power greater than yourself – a power that provides guidance and security. Faith is a deep trust in a power beyond us. This trust is ultimately translated into a belief that everything has a purpose. We may not recognize or understand that purpose, but there is a purpose in everything, even illness and suffering.

Psychosomatic illness is clear proof that the mind exerts a strong influence on our state of health and that there are variables beyond the physical symptoms of many illnesses. Even an avowed agnostic would admit that we are both physical and spiritual beings, with emotions as well as an intellect. If the two are not synchronized we can easily lose our sense of balance and perspective on life. Some refer to the spirit as the 'higher self' or the soul, and the intellect as the 'lower self' or 'personality.'

Whatever terminology we use, the fact remains that as far as an illness such as cancer is concerned, it is better if we do not try to 'go it alone.' Faith and its close relative hope are instrumental in the role our emotions play in healing. Some people have reported that they view their cancer as a gift as it confronted them with their mortality, and their cancer diagnosis was their first opportunity to explore their true nature and the meaning of their lives. In a similar way, others have stated that their cancer has, ironically, been an instrument for their healing, an opportunity to discover a source of healing and peace within, and sometimes finding that this results in a remission or cure.

The 'faith factor' has played an important part in some amazing cases of recovery from illness, although it needs to be emphasized that the chances of a physical cure by the 'faith factor' alone would be very low. There is a comprehensive set of empirical medical and psychological literature in the journals which demonstrate that religious commitment ('religious' having a broad, comprehensive definition) has a positive impact on recovery from all kinds of illness, including cancer, and that patients who adopt spiritual resources have a higher survival rate.

One of the clearest discussions on the 'faith factor' in healing is found in Dr. Bernie Siegel's best-selling book, *Love, Medicine and Miracles*. He speaks of four faiths being crucial to recovery from serious illness: faith in oneself, one's doctor, one's treatment and having spiritual faith. It is interesting that Dr. Siegel regards one's spiritual faith as the most important of all. By 'spirituality' he means acceptance, faith, forgiveness, peace and love. It is even more interesting that Siegel claims that these characteristics always appear in those who achieve unexpected healing from a serious illness such as cancer. The wonderfully reassuring thing is that hope and faith are freely available to each of us.

Dr. Carl Simonton, author of *Getting Well Again*, writes incisively about the 'faith factor' for those in need of healing:

The role of spiritual beliefs in stress management has been, to me, virtually ignored, and it's huge. Our beliefs about our nature, our beliefs about the creative forces in the universe, our beliefs about the meaning of life, our beliefs about the meaning of death – all have a huge impact on the way we live our lives. We can explore our beliefs in these areas in the same way that we can explore our beliefs about anything else, and we can determine a relative health value. And especially for people dealing with serious illness, where death is a real probability, coming to terms with issues of death is very important for freeing up energy to live.

HOPE AND LOVE – THE ANTIDOTE
TO DEPRESSION AND DESPAIR

A cancer diagnosis brings with it emotional turmoil. Even with a well-defined and long-established spirituality and strong emotional support, it took me quite a time to regain my perspective on life and to restore my sense of hope. In the months, and thankfully now years, since my diagnosis I have experienced the healing power of love and have seen its beneficial influence on others. Dr. Bernie Siegel's books on the subject, *Love, Medicine and Miracles*, and *Peace, Love and Healing* are indicative of how potent this emotion is in the healing process. At most cancer support groups you can feel that the power of love and acceptance is an integral part of the emotional support. If you visit a healing ministry service of a church, you will also have a sense of wellness because of the loving support that is yours to take. If you have a pet, your sense of wellness is enhanced because of the unconditional love it gives you. The fact is that love heals.

In what ways, then, does giving and receiving love actually heal? It strengthens our immune system. In producing endorphins, love energizes and promotes a feeling of well-being, thus enhancing our quality of life. Love is a wonderful antidote to fear. An American physician, Dr. Gerald Jampolsky, has written a book on this very subject *Love is Letting Go of Fear*.

31

Fear is the most frequently recurring (and potentially crippling) emotion I have faced since my diagnosis. Each time I have a CT scan, each time I have a blood test for my tumor marker, each time I feel unwell, I fear that the course of my illness may take a downward turn and the words of the doctor shortly after my first diagnosis echo in my ear, 'There is not a great deal we can do for your kind of mesothelioma beyond monitoring your condition.' Fear is such a naturally occurring emotion and its only antidote is faith, love and a positive mindset.

Love contributes greatly to an enhanced quality of life as it helps to relieve anxiety. It has much to do with forgiveness and forgiving, which is, in itself, healing. One writer has said that our only real protection against the uncertainties and unpredictability of life is our capacity to love and to accept love. It is the only thing that makes us feel safe and secure, whatever our outward circumstances.

In *Love, Medicine and Miracles*, Dr. Siegel states that many cancer patients have grown up believing that they have some flaw, a defect and that they are in some ways unlovable. They tend to be introverts, loners who set up defenses against sharing their innermost feelings with anyone. He writes:

When I can get people to accept themselves as whole individuals, lovable as they are, they become able to give from an inner strength. They find that unconditional love does not subtract from some limited emotional storehouse. Instead it multiplies itself. It feels good to give. It makes the recipient feel good, and sooner or later it returns...one of the immediate rewards is a 'live' message to the body. I am convinced that unconditional love is the most powerful stimulant of the immune system.

This unconditional love to which Dr. Siegel refers is not only towards oneself but to others. We need to stop being judgmental and critical and to be able to accept people as they are. We need to remember that loving, like most things in life, is a choice. It is not easy to change from being easily critical of ourselves and others to an attitude of acceptance and understanding. Remember that love and healing are always possible, irrespective of whether or not a cure takes place.

Faith, hope and love are virtually synonymous with peace, joy and optimism. All the researchers in the emerging field of mind–body medicine (psychoneuroimmunology) are suggesting that the mind and the body are one. The far-reaching implications of this fact are discussed in the next chapter.

EXERCISES TO PROMOTE FAITH AND HOPE

There is a short exercise that I have found very therapeutic and helpful in promoting faith and hope and for releasing fear, guilt, resentment and other negative mindsets that tend to impede the healing process. Their simplicity should not make you think that they are not capable of being very effective. They can only be of benefit if they are practiced on a regular daily basis. (However, do not feel guilty if through circumstance you miss a day.) They need take only fifteen to twenty minutes, although, of course, you may choose to practice them for longer. I use two famous Christian texts, St. Francis of Assisi's Peace Prayer and Psalm 23 (see Appendix Three) but you can choose whatever prayer, poem or prose that you consider promotes the same sense of calm and peace.

In order to do this exercise you will need to record the words of your choice onto an audiotape, or ask a family member or friend to do this for you. As you record these poems, take a lengthy pause between each verse. This is important. As an optional extra you might like to have soft, gentle music in the background. Then do the following:

- Choose a room where you won't be disturbed – one in which you feel safe and secure. Take the phone off the hook.

- Choose a comfortable chair. (You can do this exercise lying down, but you are less likely to fall asleep if you are sitting.) Place your feet flat on the floor, have your back reasonably straight and your head upright, or supported by the back of the chair. If you are sitting in an armchair, rest your arms on the arms of the chair; otherwise, rest your arms and hands on your thighs or loosely cupped in your lap.

- Make sure that you are comfortable, but not too comfortable. In other words, be conscious of poise and balance.

- Slowly close your eyes. Take a few slow, deep breaths. At the end of each out-breath repeat the word 'peace' in your mind. If you are feeling tense and your mind is teeming with thoughts, then just stay in this phase for a few minutes. You may wish to focus your mind on noticing or 'watching' your breath entering and leaving your nostrils.

- Switch on the cassette player. Breathe in at the beginning of each verse, as if you are breathing in its richness and beauty. Follow each verse in your mind. Affirm the truth of every verse because that is exactly what Psalm 23 is – a series of wonderful affirmations and promises. Note that these statements are made in the present tense, in the 'here and now.' The same is true of the way that St. Francis's prayer ends. Psalm 23 is among the most reassuring utterances you can ever hear. The Peace Prayer, on the other hand, is an extraordinarily powerful promise of release from everything in us that is negative, harmful to our peace of mind, and, therefore, our healing.

- When these verses have finished, sit quietly for a few minutes. If thoughts start to distract you (as they often will), focus on the breath – just 'watching' it as you did before you began the exercise.

- Finally, bring your attention back to the room and when you're ready, open your eyes. If you practice this meditative exercise regularly, eventually you will not need the tape.

Remember that faith is not a 'feel-good' state of delusion. Faith is all about releasing us from the destructive effects of negative emotions. It is abandoning fear, guilt and resentment. Faith accompanies hope. You do not need hope to believe that the sun will rise in the morning. You acknowledge this fact by faith. In the same way, you can have total faith that you can find inner healing, whatever your diagnosis or prognosis may be. Although it might be difficult to accept, inner healing is of even greater value than finding a "magic-bullet" to cure your illness.

THE POWER OF POSITIVE THINKING

These are the words of the world-famous title of the best-selling book written by Norman Vincent Peale in the 1950's. The publication of this book had a deep influence on psychology and theology in the second half of the twentieth century. New schools of 'self-empowerment' came into vogue. Some have stayed with us. In no area does the phrase "self-empowerment" have greater meaning than for sufferers of a chronic or life-threatening illness. In the 1990's a new branch of medicine dealing with the mind–body connection was formed. Various medical techniques such as biofeedback have been developed in recent years that are based on the power of the mind to heal. The philosophy of mind–body medicine is largely predicated on the fact that when we change our belief systems, our bodies possess an amazing ability to heal themselves.

In 1979, Norman Cousins, an American newspaper editor, wrote a book called *Anatomy of an Illness*. In it, Cousins described the way he had recovered from a chronic and debilitating illness he had been diagnosed with in 1964 (ankylosing spondylitis). *Anatomy of an Illness* was the story of the ways in which his doctor helped him take responsibility for his illness and mobilize his own natural healing resources. It was a landmark book in that for the first time a patient had written about the way the mind can be harnessed to help overcome disease. It remained on the United States bestseller list for over forty weeks. Cousins was keenly aware that negative emotions and tensions such as stress, frustration and anger had harmful effects on the body. The question in Cousins' mind was whether positive thoughts and emotions such as hope and optimism, joy and laughter could also alter the body's chemistry, but in a positive way. His 'experiment' ultimately worked and he eventually beat the odds and recovered from his illness. Cousins summed up his recovery in the following way:

The belief system represents the unique element in human beings that makes it possible for the human mind to affect the workings of the body.

How one responds intellectually, emotionally or spiritually to one's problems has a great deal to do with the way the human body functions. One's confidence or lack of it, in the prospects of recovery from serious illness affects the chemistry of the body. We must learn never to underestimate the capacity of the human mind and body to regenerate, even when the prospects seem most wretched...what the patient expects to happen can be as potent in touching off the biochemical processes as any medication.

In the years since Cousins wrote those words there has been a revolution in mind–body medicine. Scientific research has verified Cousins' intuitions and his experience in overcoming illness using the power of the mind. There seems to be unanimous agreement that healthy thinking enhances the body's capacity to heal. What we think and how we feel are often closely related. What follows are some practical hints on how to embrace positive attitudes and shed negativity. Being positive requires a shift in our belief systems. This is an important point made by Ian Gawler, who recovered from 'terminal' cancer, in his book *You Can Conquer Cancer*. For example, you cannot allow yourself to believe a doctor's bleak prognosis. When you choose to believe that the doctor is wrong you are enhancing your capacity to recover. You are telling your body that it will recover. You are giving your body a 'live' message. Gawler is one of many writers who state that those cancer patients who have a positive attitude, who have a strong will to live, do just that.

HOW TO 'BE POSITIVE'

It is a big challenge to 'keep your chin up' when you regularly go for blood tests, x-rays, CT scans and other unpleasant tests. Being told to be positive under these circumstances can be meaningless and even counter-productive. I recall sitting in the waiting room of the outpatients' section of the oncology unit in a large Sydney public hospital not very long after my own diagnosis. The environment was impersonal, bewildering, gloomy and certainly anything but conducive to healing or to 'being positive.' This is an all-too familiar scenario. The only possible response to this set of circumstances is in the 'faith factor,' in learning to let go of anger, guilt, fear, vulnerability, even jealousy, and to embrace loving thoughts and affirmations that anchor you in the present and prevent you from projecting those emotions into the future.

As already mentioned, hope is a potent ingredient in staying optimistic. Hope springs from your belief that tomorrow will be a better day and that your treatment can be modified or enhanced by complementary therapies. You can also enhance the power of hope by focusing on the positive aspects that have happened, and are happening, despite any setbacks. Other things you can do to stay positive include:

- RECOGNISE THAT EACH TIME YOU HAVE A SETBACK, THERE IS ALWAYS SOMETHING POSITIVE THAT HAPPENS. Think life-giving thoughts. Accentuate the positives and try eliminating the negatives. Even when outward circumstances are not good, be determined to quell the self-pity, the rage and any other self-destructive feelings that threaten your peace of mind.

- AS YOU TAKE TIME TO SIT IN QUIETNESS AND MEDITATE OR PRAY EACH MORNING AND NIGHT,

REPEAT AN AFFIRMATION ALOUD. A commonly used affirmation is 'Every day and in every way I am getting better and better.' Other suggested affirmations include: 'The Lord is my Shepherd, there is nothing that I lack'; and 'I deserve to be radiantly healthy; with every breath I feel more alive.'

- USE AFFIRMATIONS TO COUNTERACT NEGATIVITY BY REAFFIRMING THE POSITIVE. For example, if you are feeling unwell due to your treatment, affirm that: 'Each day the treatment is making me better and better.' Make sure that your affirmations are always said in the present and not in the future tense. Start or end your day with affirmations. They are a useful way of programming your belief system to affirm your healing. Use affirmations to negate the fearful effects of a difficult situation such as a particular treatment.

- AFFIRMATIONS ARE NOT EXERCISES IN WISHFUL THINKING. Rather they are a simple way of affirming your belief in your own healing. They are a recognition of your optimism.

- GIVE PRIORITY TO TIMES OF STILLNESS. This is so important because of its calming effect. We are giving ourselves much needed time-out when our minds can cease their constant chatter and we can hear our intuitive voices telling us that all will be well.

- TAKE TIME FOR A LAUGH EACH DAY. Humor is very therapeutic. This is documented in medical literature. Laughing sends endorphins through our systems and gives us a feeling of wellness, irrespective of what our medical conditions happen to be.

- BELIEVE THAT YOU HAVE THE CAPACITY TO HEAL; that tomorrow will be a better day; that each day healing is taking place and that ultimately you will win the battle.

- LEARN TO PERSEVERE WITH YOUR AFFIRMATIONS, YOUR PRAYERS, YOUR HOPE AND OPTIMISM, YOUR TIMES OF SILENCE. None of these things will reap much benefit if they are done at isolated intervals. It is very important that you establish a daily pattern where you incorporate these things into your routine.

- VISUALISE YOUR WELLNESS.

- REMEMBER THAT OUR ONLY REAL PROTECTION AGAINST THE UNCERTAINTIES OF LIFE IS OUR CAPACITY TO LOVE AND RECEIVE LOVE. Having a pet such as a dog provides a powerful lesson in unconditional love. Love quite literally can heal.

- BE ANCHORED IN THE PRESENT. The famous Russian novelist Leo Tolstoy once said, 'Now is the only time over which we have dominion.' Another writer said, 'Every situation, properly perceived, becomes an opportunity to heal.' To make these words your own will help you travel on your healing journey. To comprehend the present moment is to touch eternity, because the present moment is all we have. This should greatly help us to accept the present, whatever the prevailing circumstance.

- COMING TO TERMS WITH YOUR MORTALITY. One of the blocks to healing is the fear of death, which understandably can, and often is, a lingering fear for those with a life-threatening illness. I vividly recall the session called 'Death and Dying' at a ten-day 'Living Well' seminar that my wife and I attended at the Gawler Foundation in Victoria, Australia, soon after I was diagnosed. The reaction of a number of the participants to this 'taboo' subject was quite disturbing, in that some of the people present seemed unable to come to terms with their own mortality at a time when they were very ill and this issue pressed in on them. One person who was obviously very ill was in a state of strong denial. He was not prepared to talk about the possibility that his life could shortly be coming to a close. It was clearly evident that he had a deep fear of death. A couple of the other participants also seemed to be too tethered to their fears to be able to realize that the focus of the session was not on death itself, but on how to come to terms with our mortality and live accordingly. Whether we live another day, another month, another year, another twenty, or even more, the pertinent fact is that we should live each day we have to the full. Paradoxically, one of the ways in which cancer is a wake-up call is that it is a reminder to 'number our days' and live well.

Ian Gawler, in his book *You Can Conquer Cancer*, makes a simple but quite profound comment on death and dying:

...people often express concern about whether a particular patient should concentrate on dying well, or still be aiming to recover. In my experience, patients always seem to have this built-in instinct that directs them to concentrate on techniques for helping them in dying. Can you believe that when they are open, free of fear, those techniques are one and the same? They both aim for wholeness.

The evening we discussed this topic at the seminar the mood at the beginning was strained, especially because it was fairly obvious that some of those in the room had only a short time left to live. Yet as the session progressed, we talked openly about death and dying as if the fear, the mystery and the dread about the topic had fallen away. We even had a few laughs (amid the tears) as we discussed the rather strange wishes some of us had about how we wanted our bodies disposed of, or how we wanted our family and friends to celebrate our passing. Talking honestly and openly about death and dying and sharing our fears with each other brought a sense of release and helped us to come to terms with the fact that death is very much a part of living. If this is a subject that causes you distress, seek the help of a professional counselor. Only by talking through your fears will you be able to find release from them.

A well-known holistic doctor and author in the United States, Dr. Andrew Weil, wrote a best-selling book some years ago called *Spontaneous Healing*. In one of the chapters on healing (not on death or dying), he included a sub-heading 'Is it possible to die in a healed condition?' His answer was as follows:

Why not? Death and healing are not opposites. To die as a healed person would mean being able to view one's life as complete and accept the disintegration of the physical body. There are many reliable accounts of the last days of the sages, especially in the Buddhist traditions and extending up to the present day, that illustrate the possibility of healing into death. They bear little resemblance to what goes on in modern hospitals, where doctors often see death as the ultimate enemy to be fought with all the weapons of modern medical technology. Trapped on this battleground, patients usually have no opportunity for final healing, nor do people in our culture have ready access to practical information about using life to prepare for death...

Weil's argument that death is not the ultimate failure is very convincing. His words inspire us to see healing in its broadest perspective. They help us lift the veil of mystery and dread that our society attaches to death and dying.

MAKE FORGIVENESS A HABIT

One of the negative emotions that consumes much energy and blocks the ability to heal is resentment and inability to let go of the pains and hurts of the past. Resentment and bitterness can be directed inwardly upon ourselves, as well as towards others. Lack of forgiveness means clinging to these destructive hurts and pains. Forgiveness is sometimes the missing key to wellness. Dr. Candace Pert, in her book *Molecules of Emotion*, explains the complex interaction between the neuropeptides and the body's endocrine system. This is the interface between our emotions and our feeling of wellbeing or otherwise. When we are beset by cancer it is very important that our mindsets are focused on the healing power of love, not on fear. Only then can we hope to attain peace of mind and only then will all the other negative emotions be cancelled.

To forgive is to let go of the past, to drop all our unwanted emotional baggage, especially resentments, and feelings of guilt and bitterness. We need to accept ourselves as we are. We need to avoid judgmental attitudes and behavior, and to realize and accept that all of us are imperfect. We can accept imperfection without having to approve of it. Our expectations are often disappointed – this is part of our daily existence. Forgiving yourself and others is at the heart of practicing the difference between acceptance and approval. The key to commencing the process of forgiveness is to avoid dragging the memories of past hurts and mistakes into the present. Make an affirmation, promise solemnly to yourself that you will let go of those hurts and live in the present moment. If necessary, seek a trained counselor to talk through these issues if you feel the need is strong enough.

Dr. Joan Borysenko, an American psychologist and one of the founding researchers of mind–body medicine, wrote a book called *Guilt is the Teacher, Love is the Lesson* about the healing power of forgiveness and compassion. The book provides valuable lessons on the 'how to' of forgiveness in difficult situations, especially when someone has hurt you. One of the most important points Borysenko makes about forgiving others is that we may, in certain circumstances, forgive a person and yet still not see her again because her hurtful behavior is unlikely to change. Forgiveness is our responsibility and may not necessarily have to do with apologies (sometimes this is too big an ask) or amends on the part of the other, as nice as these might be. At times the person who hurt us may be no longer living, but we are still occupied by hatred, bitterness and resentment that slowly eats away at our peace of mind and poisons us. In this case we are prisoners of the past. The act of forgiving frees us to focus on the present and cuts away the negative thoughts that shackle us to the past.

Are there resentments and grudges you hold against anyone? Has this been going on for a long time? How does this resentment make you feel? Is this a conscious choice? Would you like to rid yourself of this grudge?

Exercise

Sit quietly and gently close your eyes. Focus your attention on your breath. For a couple of minutes simply focus your awareness on your breath coming in through your nostrils and passing out of your nostrils. Notice the flow of your breathing and feel your body relaxing and letting go of any tension. With each outbreath, imagine that you are breathing out any tension and negativity. Continue doing this for a few more minutes. When distracting thoughts invade your mind just bring your focus back to your breathing. Your sense of wellbeing will increase with each minute as your mind and body relax.

Now bring to mind a person whom you want to forgive for any wrong he might have caused you. Think about him carefully; think about his situation; think about any pain (physical or mental) that he might be suffering. Empathize with his feelings. He might well be the victim of unfortunate circumstances. He might have caused you hurt knowingly or unknowingly. Say the following sentence out loud: '(Name of person), I forgive you totally and completely. My heart goes out to you. I forgive you.' Remain in stillness. Focus your thoughts on that person. Be resolute. Mean what you say. (Some may feel fraudulent saying these words so do not worry if this does not work first time. Perseverance will pay off.) Now feel the warmth of forgiveness. Stay with that feeling of wellness. Breathe in love and peace. When you are ready, slowly open your eyes. If you wish, you can perform this exercise to the accompaniment of soft, soothing music. Do this short exercise regularly and it will definitely bring results!

The most important thing about this exercise is to do it frequently. Do not fall into the trap of convincing yourself that it does not work. It may not work the first time, but persevere – it's worth the effort! This exercise may only go a short way to solving the problem. You may need to talk this through with a trusted person, but, in time, you will find that this exercise will help you to banish the stored-up negativity that can be damaging to your healing. It is important that we are not too harsh on ourselves; that we learn to forgive ourselves our own wrongdoings and the hurt we may have caused others. It is easy to adapt this exercise to focus on forgiving ourselves. This meditation provides a good example of the phrase, 'Your healing is within you.'

PRACTICE UNCONDITIONAL LOVING

Unconditional loving follows logically from forgiveness. As already stated, giving and receiving love strongly promotes healing. Loving is not dependent on any outward circumstance. We can choose to love now, this moment. Love is a choice. It is a choice not to 'awfulize,' not to engage in negative thinking, to leave out the 'what ifs' from our lives; to live cherishing each moment, irrespective of the circumstances. The golden rule for people who are touched by cancer, either directly or indirectly, is to replace fear with love. Love is an active, not a passive thing. It is something we need to practice, together with compassion. You need to love yourself and others; to regard people in a different way from your pre-cancer days; to live with a heightened sensitivity to those who surround you.

When our circumstances are more conducive to despair than to love, remember this is precisely the time when the question of choice arises. Allow the love given by others (even those giving you the treatment) to enfold you and send out loving thoughts to others. Love each moment that you have. Love may not bring about some miraculous hoped-for cure, but it will heal you at the deepest level. It will also reduce stress and anxiety and remove despair. One writer has said that unconditional loving is the healer, and the first object of your unconditional loving is you. Love is the harbinger of hope.

THANKFULNESS

Thankfulness and gratitude are virtues that most of us have to practice consciously. You might think that this is a strange thing to say in the midst of adverse circumstances such as a life-threatening illness. In some ways it might seem strange but the fact is that whatever our circumstances, there are always blessings we have received each day. They might be small, they might be few, or they might be plentiful, but they exist and it is good for the soul to acknowledge them. You may need to sit quietly and reflect on what these blessings are: even receiving a kind smile or a kind word while undergoing treatment is significant. Then there is the gift of life, of love, of family, of friends, of being able to appreciate the beauty around us, of the presence of a higher power in our lives (if we give this power a chance to manifest itself). Many long-term cancer survivors believe that a spirit of thankfulness and gratitude, in common with a spirit of joy, brings about biochemical changes in the body that enhance our immune function.

Despair and self-pity, or seeing nothing to be thankful for, is certainly not conducive to healing. It is only when we (even briefly) stop dwelling on our illness and look beyond them that we can hope to gain a different perspective which allows us to see the big picture. How, then, do we do this? The answer lies in the simple, small things of life. Listening to music lifts our spirits and souls to a new plane, looking out at the night sky and marveling at the incredible array of stars, going to the beach and feeling the energy of nature as the waves wash on the shore. (The sound of water lapping on the seashore can be healing.)

Gratitude transforms the experience of illness and of life itself. Gratitude or thankfulness is, if you like, looking at the world through spiritual eyes, seeing beyond the day-to-day

45

experiences that often sap our energy and leave us 'down in the dumps.' An interesting and valuable exercise you can do is to make a list, on either a daily or a weekly basis, of all the good things, the blessings, that have come your way. You may be surprised at the length of your list by the end of each week.

CHAPTER SUMMARY

- The causes of cancer can be attributed to environmental, genetic and psychological factors.

- Wellness can be experienced while living with cancer. Wellness and cancer need not be mutually exclusive.

- While stress itself does not cause cancer, there is scientific evidence to suggest that certain personality types are more prone to developing cancer. There seems to be a link between some types of cancer and emotional trauma.

- The 'faith factor' is often overlooked in healing. Developing and nurturing spirituality is an important part of the healing process.

- Hope and love improve quality of life and have physiological by-products. They promote healing and can reduce anxiety and pain. Faith, hope and love are virtually synonymous with peace, joy and optimism.

- Positive thinking works mysteriously behind the scenes to help you stay well and to heal. There are exercises we can practice which encourage positive thinking.

- It is important to come to terms with our mortality. Death and healing are not opposites. Death is not a failure. Not living each day fully and lovingly is a lost opportunity. Death and dying are not taboo; they are part of life.

- Forgiveness, letting go of the past and leaving behind unwanted emotional baggage will help you towards true healing.

- Practice unconditional love. It is a vital part of the healing process and helps to allay our fears.

- Practice daily (well at least weekly) acts of gratitude and thankfulness. By doing so, you will look at the world through spiritual eyes. You will be helped to look beyond yourself and be helped to view your life in a wider perspective.

ಹಿ 3 ಡ

THE ROLE OF THE
MIND IN HEALING

THIS TOPIC MAY SEEM SLIGHTLY UNUSUAL IN A SELF-HELP BOOK FOR THOSE WHO ARE LIVING WITH CANCER. Some may regard it as too vague and theoretical. Others may wonder why their doctors do not place any emphasis on the power of the mind to promote healing. Surely the answer is that the mind, by itself, could not change the course of our illness. However, some physicians and researchers are beginning to believe that the mind exerts a far greater influence on our health than has previously been conceded. Back in the mid-1980's for example, Dr. Dean Ornish, an American heart specialist, came to the conclusion that a vegetarian diet in combination with yoga-based stretching and group support can lessen the effects of angina symptoms and slowly reverse arterial blockage. Subsequently, the studies conducted by Ornish were published in medical journals (for example, the *Journal of the American Medical Association or JAMA*) and were confirmed by others.

The link between thoughts and the state of our health is hardly a new phenomenon. Hippocrates in ancient Greece, acknowledged as the father of medicine, suggested that good health was a balance between mind, body and the environment. The writer of the *Book of Proverbs* in the Bible stressed that 'as a man thinks, so he is.' Seventeen centuries after Hippocrates, a French philosopher, Descartes, wrote that the mind, body and spirit were separate entities. Modern medicine has tended to follow Descartes' line of thinking. The focus of modern medical practice has often been on curing the symptoms and ignoring the underlying causes of illness.

In recent years there has been a growing interest in mind–body medicine. Books, magazine articles and television and radio documentaries have been suggestive of this interest. Dr. Andrew Weil's book *Spontaneous Healing* drew the public's attention to some profound truths about the mind–body connection. Weil made the point that the majority of those in the medical profession do not take mind–body medicine seriously. Therefore, research funds are not allocated to this branch of medicine and what research does exist is often of poor quality. Weil is one of the increasing number of doctors who practice a model of health and healing predicated on mind–body interaction. His clinical experience has taught him to take seriously the correlation between mental/emotional events and healing responses. He says 'These correlations are important because they suggest ways that people can keep their healing systems in good working order and can use their minds to promote healing rather than obstruct it.'

CHANGING YOUR BELIEFS ABOUT CANCER

It cannot be overemphasized how important it is to adopt a positive mindset when facing a life-threatening illness such as cancer. Below are five positive and helpful thoughts you can embrace to assist you in combating negativity and fear, and to help you towards healing.

- CANCER CAN BE OVERCOME. This belief is stated in the light of the many people who have survived against the odds from a whole range of cancers. There are many things you can do to help your situation – irrespective of the prognosis. This is said not to defy your doctor or to belittle or ignore their professional expertise. Rather, this belief is stated because your doctor cannot be aware of all the variables involved in your unique case. As stated in Chapter

1, your doctor's prognosis is made in the light of statistics related to your type of cancer.

- YOUR TREATMENT REGIME WILL HELP IN YOUR RECOVERY. Visualize each treatment bringing you a step closer to healing.

- EVERYTHING IN YOUR LIFE HAS A PURPOSE AND A PLAN. Unfortunately, we often cannot see or do not understand the big picture. We need to nurture spirituality in our life – to look at life beyond the 'here and now' and beyond the 'ups and downs' of our daily existence. We need to have faith that we are not the plaything of fate and fortune. We need to focus on a power beyond ourselves. By doing this we put our lives into a fuller and more meaningful context. We need to remember that we are spiritual, as well as physical beings.

- HOPE IS PHYSIOLOGICAL! Hope affects the way we feel. Hope in the form of positive beliefs affects our recovery. Our beliefs and expectations often set the course of our actual experience, not merely in the realm of a cancer diagnosis.

- TO THINK POSITIVELY IS A MATTER OF CHOICE! POSITIVE THINKING ACTUALLY WORKS. Most of our belief system is something we have inherited – something we have not consciously chosen. Our beliefs can be very powerful. Think about your beliefs. How do they help or hinder your situation?

Exercise

Think carefully for a few minutes about your cancer diagnosis. Then write down all your feelings and thoughts that come to mind in regard to your diagnosis.

- Make a list of your beliefs about your treatments.

- List the three or four things that you feel would best assist in your recovery.

- Analyze how your beliefs compared with the thoughts stated above. Talk to other cancer survivors. Find out what they believe. Make a conscious decision to change any beliefs that are self-limiting.

THE POWER OF THE MIND TO HEAL

Chapter 6 looks more closely at the beneficial healing effects of meditation, which is one way we can use our minds to help our bodies heal. As mentioned earlier, the late Dr. Ainslie Meares wrote about the therapeutic effects of meditation in a book written in beautiful verse called *Cancer: Another Way?*

For the moment, it is important to realize that choosing to have a positive mindset about your situation is an incredibly simple choice. At the same time it is a choice that you need to make deliberately and consciously. We must be like a ship sailing across the sea. Although it encounters all weathers, it does not change course in mid-voyage when the weather turns rough. We might need to increase the time we devote to meditation or prayer; we might need to reassess our treatment regime, but we cannot, we dare not change our positive mindset and allow our emotional health to suffer. Make an affirmation such as 'I am a positive person now' each morning. Repeat this affirmation aloud at various times during the day till it becomes your firm conviction. Feel positive and develop a strong belief and trust that each time you have your treatment, it is helping you to get better. (The converse of this is that if you adopt a negative attitude towards your treatment, the chances of it working will substantially decrease.)

In Chapter 2 you will find a number of other affirmations to help you confirm and strengthen your conviction and belief to stay positive. Research has shown that our beliefs do make a difference to both the quality of our life and the 'quantity' of our survival. The importance of our beliefs is graphically illustrated in the stories of those who have outlived their prognoses or those who have achieved remarkable recoveries.

Finally, remember that to aim for, what one writer has called a 'dynamic state of peace,' is absolutely paramount. In other words, if we invest all our energies in trying to bring about a cure, we are robbing ourselves of peace of mind. We are trying to live in the future and not in the present. A 'dynamic state of peace' is all about making peace of mind our first priority; working at it, as it were. This is an attainable goal; our physical cures are also vital goals that may or may not be achievable, but it is important that we have a determination to live in the present moment and not project our fears into the future. We need to give our bodies every opportunity for self-healing. A positive expectancy (or belief) in whatever treatments we are having is an important contributor to outlasting our prognoses.

THE MYSTERY OF THE PLACEBO

Most doctors would agree that a placebo – any imitation medicine that has the appearance of an authentic medication but which contains no beneficial substances at all – does actually work. The amazing thing is that it can work for almost any illness, including a life-threatening illness such as cancer. Ever since the 1960's and even earlier, researchers have been working on the connection between illness and psychological factors and the ways in which a placebo actually works in helping people to overcome the symptoms of their illness. There are many theories as to how placebos work, including one that claims that the belief that an effective drug has been taken activates the cerebral cortex of the brain, which in turn activates the endocrine system and then the adrenal glands. Placebos have the advantage that they do not have the side-effects of conventional drugs.

Norman Cousins, in *Anatomy of an Illness*, claimed that 90 percent of patients who reach out for medical help are suffering from self-limiting disorders well within the range of the body's own healing powers. The implications of this for our medical system are staggering. Equally staggering is the fact that because placebos actually work they prove that our beliefs and our hopes can be transformed into tangible changes that can be measured by the biochemical changes in our bodies. That is why we can argue that hope is physiological. The placebo illustrates that the mind and body are inextricably linked. Whether illness begins in the body and then affects the mind or vice versa, the fact is that we cannot separate these two entities.

More and more doctors are taking a holistic view of medicine, seeing mind and body as an integrated system. There is an increasing body of research showing the various ways in which the mind and body are one. Scientists such as Dr. Robert Ader of the University of Rochester in the United States are demonstrating how our emotional states can alter our hormonal profiles, which can influence our blood chemistry, heart rates and immune functions. Dr. Ader was featured in a popular American television series some years ago called 'Healing and the Mind,' with Bill Moyers. Ader's chief interest was to study the neurological and hormonal impact of stress on the immune system. More specifically, he wanted to find out how our emotional states affect our nervous system and how those in combination affect our immune systems. His work on rats produced some amazing results, including the fact that he actually conditioned the immune function of rats by using various behavioral modification techniques based on Pavlovian experiments. Ader is one of a number of scientists worldwide who are breaking new ground in the field of psychoneuroimmunology. 'Psycho' refers to mind, thoughts, emotions; 'neuro' refers to the nervous system; 'immunology' having to do with the immune system.

Psychoneuroimmunology studies the effects of our thoughts and emotions on our bodies' susceptibility or resistance to disease. Another leading scientist in this field is Dr. Candace Pert, also from the United States. She dropped a bombshell into conservative medical circles by suggesting that the findings of psychoneuroimmunology, or mind–body medicine render the conceptual division between the sciences of immunology, endocrinology and psychology as a historical artifact. Her argument is documented in her groundbreaking book *Molecules of Emotion*. In this book, Dr. Pert explains the existence of a communicating network of neuropeptides and their receptors that provides a link among the body's cellular defense and repair mechanisms, glands and brain.

To date, relatively few doctors have taken much notice of mind–body medicine and the possibility that it can impact a patient's chances of recovery. This is not an area that most physicians have studied during their medical education, so it is not surprising that they do not take it seriously. However, more and more doctors are realizing that physical treatment alone can provide only limited benefits. It seems that cases of remarkable recovery beg to find answers from a biomedical model. Neurophysiologists such as Pert and others have established a link between the brain and the immune system. This link is a further reason to believe that the patient must believe in her doctor and the treatment being received in order for recovery to be enhanced.

Regardless of how we are put together psychologically, we are all going to die from something. It is a fact that many saintly people from various faiths have died of cancer. It would be crass to suggest that they died because of unhealed emotional problems or because they were unable to achieve peace of mind. We need to realize that on this side of the grave there are questions that cannot be answered. Life does indeed have mysterious elements. We cannot afford to see someone who has lost the fight against cancer as having been a failure. Rather, we should see such a case in its fullest perspectives.

Dr. Larry Dossey wrote a book called *Recovering the Soul – A Scientific and Spiritual Search*. One aspect of this fascinating book is a call to his medical colleagues to realize that it is not possible to look at medicine, psychology and spirituality as separate disciplines. Like Dr. Pert, he states that the mind is not just the brain but part of a wider network. He quotes Albert Einstein who once said that it is a 'delusion of our consciousness' to suggest that our brain is just a phenomenon of nervous activity.

The above discussion suggests that an illness such as cancer is a reminder that we have a spiritual dimension that needs nurturing, just as our physical bodies need nurturing and care. The issue of suffering is so broad as to be mostly beyond the scope of this book. However, a few appropriate words about this subject are necessary because it is a topic that is intrinsic to a life-threatening illness such as cancer.

The experience of suffering can easily lure us into a mindset of being a victim. 'Why me?' The way we view suffering is to a large extent dependent on the way we view the rest of life. For some, suffering becomes meaningless and completely cruel without a spiritual framework to life. Personally, I find that mental and spiritual pain is harder to handle than physical pain, which can be more readily controlled. However, peace of mind can be achieved while still not having controlled one's symptoms or having halted or reversed one's illness, for peace of mind is to a large extent dependent on being emotionally healthy. Even suffering can be seen in a positive way. It can teach us compassion and the value of unconditional love. Suffering can be part of the 'wake-up call' of a cancer diagnosis and healing journey. In other words, it can heighten our awareness of our spiritual dimension and jolt us into a reality beyond our humdrum daily existence. It is amazing the number of cancer patients, especially long-term survivors, who say that their cancer diagnosis turned out to be positive because they now live much more purposeful lives.

The experience of cancer helps us to see that the real treasures of life are not to be found in the externals but in inner peace and contentment. Suffering is, not unnaturally, closely related to the 'faith factor' discussed in the last chapter. All of us experience suffering at some time in our lives. The critical issue is how we respond to it. What follows is intended to help us to

55

see illness (not just cancer) in a different (and hopefully, more meaningful) light.

ADOPTING A MINDSET FOR BECOMING A LONG-TERM SURVIVOR

Dr. Siegel has written a great deal about the critical importance of attitude as a determinant of surviving cancer. Most of his many books are variations of this theme, and it is the recurring theme in the stories about cancer survivors. Dr. Siegel would often ask his cancer patients four questions. Siegel claimed that the answers his patients gave to these questions were a reliable indicator of their chances of recovery. He would ask:

- 'Do you want to live to be 100?'
- 'What does this illness mean to you?'
- 'Why did you need this illness?'
- 'What happened in the year or so before your diagnosis?'

In response to whether or not you want to be 100, Siegel claimed that the answer gave him an idea whether or not his patients felt in control of their lives and whether they looked forward to the future. The answer to the second question was an indicator as to whether the person saw the illness as a challenge to overcome or as an overwhelming obstacle – a virtual death sentence. The answer revealed to Siegel whether the person had made the prognosis a part of his belief system. In other words, it revealed whether or not the prognosis had filtered down into the subconscious mind. The answer to the third question reveals whether or not the disease serves some psychological or emotional purpose. It might be a plea for love or nurturing or it might be a plea for some time out. The final question is asked to elicit whether or not some major change or challenge had occurred recently in their lives. Siegel claimed that very commonly a person had undergone some change, or had experienced a crisis that could have suppressed immune function.

In *Peace, Love and Healing*, Siegel leaves no doubt that the patients who give themselves the maximum opportunity to heal are those who view their cancer as messages to redirect their lives. These are people who resolve conflicts with others and are able to express the emotions they have been bottling up inside (sometimes for years). Furthermore, they are people who stop ignoring their own needs and learn to love themselves, as well as others. As I have already indicated, attitude, or one's mindset, is a powerful stimulus to physical health and for long-term survival. This is why emotional healing is important in order to come to terms with a life-threatening illness such as cancer.

YOUR EMOTIONS ARE CHEMICAL

Dr. Candace Pert's book *Molecules of Emotion* is subtitled *The Science Behind Mind–Body Medicine*, indicating an explanation of the physiological basis of emotions, or to use her term, the 'molecular underpinnings of what we experience as feelings, sensations, thoughts, drives, perhaps even spirit or soul.'

Pert devotes much of her book to explaining the mechanisms of the role of the mind in healing. For example, several of her chapters discuss the operations of the autonomic nervous system, the way neurotransmitters, hormones and growth regulators work. She notes that receptors for many of the neurotransmitters cluster in the gut and in the brain, especially in areas concerned with emotion. Many of the receptors in the gut are endorphin receptors. She says that there is indeed a biochemical meaning to the term 'gut feeling', suggesting that our gut is also a seat of emotion. Since cells of the immune system have receptors for many of these peptide molecules, it is likely that our defenses are also part of the interconnecting network linking our nervous systems and our endocrine systems. To express Pert's argument in non-scientific terms, our emotions can have a significant impact on our bodies at the cellular level. It is, of course, at the cellular level that a disease such as cancer works.

Therefore, the way we respond to our illness could not only determine our quality of life but also our quantity of life. Unfortunately, the mind–body aspects of healing, when applied to cancer, remain in the shadows because of the economics and politics of cancer. Psychoneuroimmunology is not well established in orthodox medicine. It is not in the best interest of drug companies, for whom cancer is a multi-billion dollar industry, to be convinced that their products may not always be the most suitable therapy for certain types of cancer. Fortunately, some physicians are beginning to acknowledge the role of the mind in healing and are using therapies and treatments that take this important factor into account.

WHAT ARE EMOTIONS?

The term 'emotion' can be interpreted to include not only the familiar human experiences of anger, fear and sadness, but also pleasure and pain. This is a broad and somewhat loose definition, probably rejected by some scientists who argue, for example, that things like temperament are genetic as much as psychological. Nevertheless, what we commonly understand as emotions, are usually limited to either positive or negative feelings that we experience in our everyday lives. However, there are other intangible, subjective experiences that are probably unique to humans – experiences such as spiritual inspiration, awe, bliss and other states of consciousness that we have all experienced but that have been, up until now, physiologically unexplained.

Dr. Pert's chapter 'The Biochemicals of Emotion,' in her book *Molecules of Emotion*, is an explanation of the way in which our thoughts influence the functioning of our bodies, in particular, the functioning of our immune systems. There is a steadily mounting body of evidence suggesting that stress, in its various manifestations, can be a causative factor in cancer. The rather simplistic notion that what is in your mind will eventually affect your body is explored in some detail by Dr. Pert. She says that many of the mind–body interactions take place at the subconscious level. We can visualize the blood flow increasing to a body part, for example, and that will indeed happen. The way we think and feel, consciously or unconsciously, can alter a number of our physiological states. Psychological studies have been conducted to show the truth of this argument. Some years ago, for example, a study of hospital patients who stayed in a bright, airy ward with a view of lovely gardens showed that their healing responses were significantly more rapid than another group of patients whose only view to the outside was a brick wall. The medically accepted therapy of biofeedback is based solely on the mind–body interaction.

The body, right down at the cellular level, is heavily influenced by the level of our emotional health. It is amazing to think that such 'awareness' or 'intelligence' (for example, how many white cells to produce) can be located at the cellular level! That is precisely why Dr. Pert called her book *Molecules of Emotion*. When reading accounts of those who have had remarkable recoveries from cancer I have wondered about the extent to which they achieved their recoveries through 'self-induced healing.' People do become empowered to heal through utilizing positive emotions (such as faith, hope, love and laughter) together with adopting healthy, carefully disciplined lifestyles. So many times I see people who do not have healthy lifestyles in terms of such usual yardsticks as nutrition and exercise, yet they do not succumb to life-threatening illnesses such as heart disease or cancer. Genetic factors may help explain why this happens but I am convinced that a happy disposition also plays a role.

I have found, both from my own experience and that of my fellow cancer sufferers that one of the biggest stumbling blocks to healing is a reluctance to let go of our fears and our negative ways of thinking. Faith is a paradox. It is essentially a simple thing – a matter of complete trust and a strongly held belief. Yet, we are often unwilling to grasp a particular belief, or a strong hope. Why? Because we seem unwilling to accept anything that is not tangible. The very simplicity of having a childlike faith is its greatest stumbling block. Faith and hope are not synonymous with wishful thinking. From the above discussion on the mind–body connection we can argue that when faith and hope are embraced, they are translated into tangible healing benefits.

The commencement of my own journey with cancer illustrates this truth. Conventional treatment had little to offer. The only way forward, for the time being, was to monitor my condition. This worried me deeply. I changed my lifestyle and diet. As the days turned into weeks I felt that valuable time was being wasted and began to feel rather desperate about the situation. My reaction was to seek out a number of other opinions. My desperation for answers increased with the passing of time. It took a while to realize that the radical change of lifestyle upon which I had embarked was in itself a form of treatment. The liters of carrot and green juices I was daily consuming, the array of nutritional supplements I was taking, the daily meditation and prayer was my treatment and was aiding my body to recover. The problem was that I had been so conditioned to believe that if the treatment was not conventional then it was second-rate. I found it enormously difficult to 'let go and let God' probably because my faith in God under testing times was weak.

HOW YOU CAN USE YOUR
MIND TO PROMOTE HEALING

Observe your emotions and acknowledge them – not merely the positive emotions such as faith, hope and love – but the so-called negative ones such as anger and guilt. Do not bottle them up and deny them lest they ultimately overwhelm you. Denying your emotions is not conducive to healing. Try to find someone with whom you can talk, possibly a trained counselor, or at least a good friend in whom you can safely confide. Remember, your emotions are chemical. They can either help to balance your body chemistry or they can lower your body's defenses and thereby your immune function. Medical evidence suggests that there is a correlation between our healing responses and our mental and emotional health.

- BE CONSCIOUS THAT LIFE IS ALL ABOUT CHOICES. Be aware not just of your physical welfare, but of your spirituality, your emotional experiences. Make time to be silent at various times in the day – what Dr. Bernie Siegel calls 'healing intervals' to remind yourself that you are human being, not a human doing. In doing this you will enhance your body's self-healing capacities. You will be sending 'healing messages' to your subconscious. So many of our basic bodily functions, such as breathing and digestion, happen at an autonomic or subconscious level.

- THE MIND IS HEAVILY INFLUENCED BY EMOTIONAL PEPTIDES (IN THE FORM OF CERTAIN AMINO ACID CHAINS). When we adopt a negative mindset and 'bottle up' unhealthy feelings such as resentment and guilt – some of which we have harbored for years – we can block our natural healing mechanisms. Practice the forgiveness exercise outlined in the last chapter. Regularly use affirmations (see Chapter 6), meditation and prayer to help you let go of the past and focus your awareness on the present. You may need professional help in the form of counseling to help you let go of the past, with its negativities. Do not hesitate to do this because your healing system will not function efficiently if you neglect your emotional health.

- BE AWARE OF YOUR BODY'S NEED OF EXERCISE. Exercise is an important aid in reducing stress and helping your body's self-healing mechanisms to function optimally. Walk, swim, and learn the gentle healing arts of tai chi or yoga. All of these are very healing. Practice self-honesty and personal integrity – towards others and towards yourself. It reduces stress and promotes healing.

- EAT WISELY! What we eat and the way we eat is related to our emotional states. Eating is another lifestyle choice that can be reframed in light of our understanding of the emotions. In part, this is so because physiologically the large and small intestines contain an abundance of neuropeptides and receptors. In other words, your thoughts and emotions considerably affect your digestive functions. Certain cancers are affected by the metabolism; and what we eat affects our metabolic functions. The subject of nutrition is discussed in the next chapter.

- SPIRITUALITY IS NOT REGARDED AS BEING THE DOMAIN OF THE MEDICAL PROFESSION YET ITS IMPACT ON HEALTH AND HEALING IS CONSIDERABLE. Remember, spirituality is not the same thing as 'religion,' which has doctrinal connotations and which therefore tends to divide, rather than unite people. As someone once remarked, 'We are spiritual beings in a physical body and not the other way around.' Forgiveness – forgiving oneself and others is healing. We need to be healed from negative past experiences by the art of forgiving.

- SHIFT THE FOCUS OF YOUR CONSCIOUSNESS INTO A MODE OF ACCEPTANCE, NOT CONFRONTATION. Too many of us live life in a confrontationist mode, trying to shape events or impose our wills to shape events and to control situations.

This is an excerpt taken from *Prescriptions for Living*, by Dr. Bernie Siegel.

Who or what can give you peace? Nothing but your own mind. You must live peace to experience peace. If your peace of mind depends on the world meeting your needs, you won't find peace very often. When you do, it won't last ... More often, life presents you with difficulties. A lasting peace will never come until you change your mind about what you need, and learn the difference between what you want and what you need ... True peace comes when you have faith. That peace depends not on external events but on the state of your mind. You are the source and the recipient ... If you have faith you will RIP the rest of your lifetime.

Please remember that everything about the role of the mind in healing is directed towards helping to heal. This extends far beyond your cancer diagnosis. This subject is firstly, all about enhancing the quality of your life and, in turn, hopefully extending its quantity also.

CHAPTER SUMMARY

- Health and healing – both physical and emotional – are dependent on a balance between mind, body and the environment. The way we think determines the way we act.

- Do not 'awfulize' your cancer diagnosis, rather imprint positive, 'live' messages into your subconscious mind, for example, that cancer can, and has been, overcome.

- It is a simple choice to think positively, whatever the doctors say about your prognosis. Doctors are only human and they have been known to err, especially when it comes to predicting the course of an individual's illness.

- Mind–body medicine, or psychoneuroimmunology, is gathering more and more scientific evidence that there is a close link between mind and body. Your immune function is affected by your emotional health.

- Emotionally healthy people and deeply spiritual people can, and do, get cancer. This is but one of many variables for having a 'predisposition' for this illness.

- The 'mind' is part of an enormously complex network. The mind is not just the brain.

- A cancer diagnosis is often a wake-up call that we are spiritual as well as physical beings. We need to take this dimension of our being seriously and live accordingly.

- Suffering has an ultimate purpose – mysterious as this may seem. 'The darker the night of suffering, the more radiant the life of pure love that emerges from it,' said a nineteenth century writer.

- Your body, even at the cellular level, has an incredible capacity for self-healing. Your 'molecules of emotion' scientifically described by Dr. Candace Pert are one proof of this.

- Faith and hope are not synonymous with wishful thinking. They are real for you. They have physiological side effects!

- Regularly try the meditation exercise on forgiveness and compassion. You will gain much benefit from it. These qualities also have tangible benefits for the healing process.

ಖ 4 ଙ

CONVENTIONAL AND COMPLEMENTARY THERAPIES

THERE ARE A NUMBER OF ASSUMPTIONS, MYTHS AND CONSTRAINTS REGARDING CANCER TREATMENTS – BOTH CONVENTIONAL AND UNCONVENTIONAL. The terms 'alternative' or 'complementary' therapies can be confusing. An alternative therapy is one that is not supplied or officially approved of by conventional medicine. They can vary from the well known such as acupuncture, osteopathy, naturopathy and herbal to the lesser used such as Bach flower remedies and reiki. Many people choose to complement their conventional treatments with some form of therapy not provided by their doctors. Complementary therapies, as the name suggests, are in addition to conventional or orthodox cancer treatments. They include all forms of therapy that fall outside the conventional forms of cancer treatment. The terms 'complementary' and 'alternative' treatments can overlap. Recent studies in mainstream medical journals such as *The Journal of Oncology* demonstrate that the majority of cancer patients are now using some form of alternative or complementary therapy. Why is this happening? The answer is worth considering.

Medical science acknowledges that there is no universal cure for cancer. Conventional treatments have their limitations and, in certain cancers, especially those that have spread or metastasized, have extremely limited success. Surgery still seems to be the most effective conventional method of removing tumors. Providing the cancer has not spread widely, surgery can have a high rate of success. The next line of defense is chemotherapy and radiation, which aim to shrink tumors. However, the success rate of both chemotherapy and radiation in bringing about complete remission is, for most types of cancer, still relatively low. Further, these therapies are toxic and, in some cases have unpleasant side effects that can significantly reduce quality of life.

Despite these limitations, many medical practitioners hold some hostility towards alternative or complementary cancer treatments. This is understandable because of the danger of a patient following an altogether unproven treatment given by an unscrupulous therapist, probably at considerable cost. At the same time, the orthodox doctor may not realize that there are many self-help techniques that one can adopt that are beneficial for wellness and that will help heal.

In some ways the divide between conventional 'scientific' and the 'non-scientific' complementary cancer treatments is unfortunate. The holistic medical philosophy, which is more prevalent in Europe than in either the United States or in Australia, emphasizes that healing must take the whole person into account – body, mind and spirit. Indeed, it is possible for a person to die in a healed state – feeling at perfect peace with herself. With the materialist and secularized viewpoint that is the norm these days, we tend to forget that we are all 'terminal' cases and that overcoming cancer does not necessarily equate with going on to live a happy or healed life. Curing cancer, or any other illness, is not the whole story of getting well again. 'Healing' is a far more inclusive term than 'curing.' This is a subject that will be covered in greater detail in the next chapter. What follows are a few words of advice to the newly diagnosed.

A naturopath, herbalist or any other natural therapist may not be permitted by law to treat cancer. The treatments they provide are usually designed to help you build and strengthen your nutritional intake so that your body's immune function will be enhanced and therefore your body will be in a better state to fight your illness. Natural therapists believe that a highly nutritious diet can help a person in their quest of getting well again, particularly when the body is stressed by such toxic treatments as chemotherapy and radiation. In addition, it is an established scientific fact that a poor diet is a contributing factor in the development of certain types of cancer. Further, if we accept the fact that cancer is a metabolic disease, then improving one's metabolic function by a very nutritious diet and dietary supplements must, by definition, be helpful. A strong argument can therefore be mounted for cancer patients (and those with other chronic illnesses) to adopt major dietary changes and to use nutritional supplementation such as vitamins, minerals, herbs and amino acids.

TREATMENT SELECTION

There are at least two problems facing cancer patients when it comes to the matter of treatment selection. The first is that at the time of diagnosis the conventional treatment options presented are often limited, particularly when the success rate is questioned. The second problem lies with advice supplied by well-intentioned family, friends and acquaintances – not to mention the Internet! There is frequently an 'information overload' and some of this information may seem contradictory, especially when it comes to the most useful forms of therapy. Be aware of who gives you the information and its source.

By far the most important advice regarding your treatment is to choose a doctor with whom you can relate well and who has wide experience in dealing with your type of cancer. They will be in the best possible position to help you. The doctor you want is someone who is able to listen to your questions and concerns and is able to you offer you hope. I do not mean 'false hope.' False hope exists only when you are given information that is untrue.

I repeat, only by willfully giving a person misleading information can a medical practitioner (or anyone, for that matter) engender false hope. A medical practitioner should have something positive to tell you beyond the statistics of your illness. This is a point I stressed in the opening chapter and its importance cannot be overstated. My surgeon left me devoid of hope. It was a terrible feeling.

The crucial thing for you to do is to make a well-informed treatment decisions. My experience has shown me that two things frequently happen following a cancer diagnosis. Firstly, it is easy to be intimidated by the initial doctor's treatment recommendations, sometimes without fully understanding the implications a treatment has on affecting a cure. Secondly, you discover that there is a whole world of alternative or complementary cancer therapies that may be beneficial. While some of these therapies may be expensive, others are not. This is another area that requires discernment.

After a diagnosis you are, above all, seeking the best possible treatment. It is natural to be attracted to anything that offers hope of a cure. Unfortunately, it is at just such a time that you are vulnerable to misinformation. Misinformation can come from the field of natural therapies or orthodox medicine. Therefore, it is important that the doctor you select is able to provide meaningful support and insight for any treatment claim regarding survival and quality of life.

CANCER THERAPY AND CULTURE

In his book *Choices in Healing*, Dr. Michael Lerner draws some interesting contrasts between the mainstream, conventional approach to cancer treatment in the United States and the approaches in various European countries, particularly Germany, the United Kingdom and France.

Lerner describes the American approach to medical treatment as 'aggressive medicine.' For example, there are more caesarean births (c-sections) in the United States than in any European country. Similarly, more people die in the hospital; more patients die from medical errors (over 100,000 year according to a Harvard study); there are more invasive diagnostic tests performed, and surgery is generally more radical than it is for comparable operations in Europe. The same trend exists in terms of cancer treatment: radical mastectomies and radical irradiation techniques are more routinely used than in Europe. The entire focus of cancer treatment is on cure by aggressively attacking the cancer, rather than on minimization or remission. The reasons for this are numerous, including the system of reimbursement in the U.S. (For many physicians, the more procedures they perform or drugs they administer, the greater their income.)

The German medical model presents a marked contrast. For example, in Germany conventional treatment is used in conjunction with adjunctive or complementary treatments. Many doctors combine chemotherapy with alternative methods of cancer treatment such as the use of herbs, especially to aid in detoxifying the body. Many others incorporate intensive use of naturopathic, homoeopathic and anthroposophic medicine (based on the spiritual principles of Rudolf Steiner and various forms of folk medicine). The German medical system has, therefore, a more holistic orientation, which takes into account a person's healing potential. There is little doubt that a German cancer patient has a much broader choice of treatments and therapies than an American.

As to the all important question of survival rates in each of these countries, there is no clear-cut answer. What is known, however, is that a cancer patient's quality of life is enhanced by having a sense of empowerment and a degree of responsibility for their illness. Also, the complementary therapies used in conjunction with conventional treatments mitigate the adverse symptoms of toxic treatments and are used to enhance the patient's immune function.

POINTS TO CONSIDER FOR CONVENTIONAL TREATMENTS

- Remember that the majority of cancers, if detected at a relatively early stage, are potentially curable. People have recovered from all types of cancer, including aggressive types such as pancreatic and lung cancer.

- If the best medical advice strongly recommends surgical removal of a tumor, then follow that advice. Statistically, surgery has been shown to have a higher success rate than any other form of conventional treatment.

- If your doctor recommends chemotherapy and radiation, first of all find out what the success rate is for that treatment for your type of cancer and for your stage of that illness. Apart from asking your oncologist, research what is published about a specific treatment on Medline www.pubmed.gov or use an online treatment database like Cancer Monthly www.cancermonthly.com that provides information on treatment results from the published medical literature.

- Refer to a medical library. Sometimes, a good local library will have reasonably detailed reference books on cancer and its treatment.

- Talk to other patients who have undergone the same treatment. They can give you a good idea what to expect.

- If you are having chemotherapy or radiation treatment, keep a close track of the recommended doses you are given each time. Monitor as best you can the course of your treatment. Practitioners have been known to make mistakes because they are so busy and work under pressure. These treatments are toxic and can cause damage to organ function.

- If you are having chemotherapy or radiation, discontinue any vitamin or mineral tablets, especially any antioxidants, such as vitamins A, C or E, as they may interfere with your treatment. However, it is important that you continue your supplements as soon as your treatment is over, as antioxidants, especially vitamin A, can protect you from side-effects and help to protect healthy cells.

POINTS TO CONSIDER FOR ALTERNATIVE/ COMPLEMENTARY TREATMENTS

- Alternative cancer therapies include some of the best and some of the worst treatments available. There are certain unconventional treatments that have been proven to enhance quality of life, promote general health, and engage patients in their treatment in psychologically and sometimes physically beneficial ways. The worst treatments are those undertaken for financial gain by unscrupulous people. Certain complementary or adjunctive treatments, such as meditation, juicing, adherence to an anti-cancer diet and herbal and/or homoeopathic treatments are increasingly being used by patients to supplement other forms of treatment they may be having.

- Many of the so-called alternative and complementary cancer treatments have healing, rather than curing, as their primary focus. Many medical practitioners (and virtually all natural therapists) would agree that the primary aim of complementary therapies is to control a person's cancer (i.e. stop it from growing) and to improve quality of life, rather than aiming at a cure (i.e. destruction of the cancer). If you want to read a comprehensive summary of the philosophy and practice of complementary cancer treatments you will find no better discussion than Chapters 7 to 10 in Lerner's *Choices in Healing.*

- The medical profession remains cynical (and often openly hostile) to complementary cancer therapies, mainly due to their lack of scientific evidence and to doctors' ignorance of their use. Although this is understandable, it is unfortunate that many doctors do not realize the psychological, spiritual, and often physical benefits to be gained by patients who use certain complementary treatments, particularly nutritional supplements, which relatively few orthodox doctors understand.

71

- Check on the credentials of the health professional from whom you are planning to receive treatment. As a starting point, make sure that the person is a member of a reputable organization of health practitioners.

- Research the alternative or complementary treatments that you are considering. For example, there is a small but steadily growing body of scientific evidence being published on complementary cancer treatments such as intravenous vitamin C. (Nobel Prize Winner Dr. Linus Pauling wrote a book on the importance of vitamin C in controlling cancer – *Cancer and Vitamin C*.) Make every effort to obtain credible information before starting on a particular course of treatment. (The Internet is a useful tool here. Also see Useful Contacts and Resources at the end of this book.)

- Ask your practitioner about any toxic side effects from the recommended therapy. If possible, speak to people who have undergone your proposed therapy.

- Whatever treatment you opt for, be aware that your body has succumbed to cancer, which means that your 'healing system,' or your immune system, has failed to do its job. Therefore, it can only be in your best interest to do everything possible to improve your overall level of health.

MONITORING TREATMENTS

How do you know that an unconventional treatment is working? Is it just because your symptoms start to recede? The only reliable way to find out is by having your condition monitored by your doctor. My regular blood tests and CT scans (together with the fact that I was continuing to feel well) was a reasonable indicator that progress was being made in halting the course of my illness.

COMMONLY USED UNCONVENTIONAL THERAPIES

Most commonly used unconventional therapies are *complementary* to conventional treatment and not alternatives to it. All these therapies, to a greater or lesser degree, may aid in healing. They all play a part in helping to mobilize the healing system, but only seldom, where medical science has nothing more to offer (as in my case), do they take the place of conventional treatment. As I have already suggested, the choices in complementary therapies are many.

Before embarking on a complementary treatment you need to ask yourself some questions. These might include:

- Can I afford to use it for as long as the treatment is recommended?

- Do I believe in this approach, or do I have doubts about its efficacy?

- Does this treatment conflict with my belief systems?

- How is this treatment monitored?

- What is its record of success?

Because most natural therapies are not easily patentable, drug companies have not invested money to bring these treatments to market. The result is that there is less data in the mainstream medical journals about the efficacy and safety of these therapies. Therefore, intuition may play a role in deciding the answers to a number of the above questions. An important consideration by cancer patients for using complementary treatments is that they are non-toxic and holistic. Of course make sure that there are no compatibility problems with any complementary and orthodox treatment that you wish to use simultaneously. This is particularly the case with taking certain vitamins.

Once you begin a treatment then go with it and cast doubts aside. Believe that this treatment is working for you. Dr. Andrew Weil, in his best-selling book *Spontaneous Remission*, emphasizes that belief in the healing power of some person, place or thing can be a key to its success. This is in the realm of the power of the mind rather than mere wishful thinking. The latter is not connected directly to the autonomic nervous system and other controlling mechanisms of the healing system.

There are five major categories of unconventional therapies used in cancer treatment: (1) nutrition and diet, (2) traditional Chinese medicine, (3) herbal medicine, (4) oxygen and ozone therapy, and (5) pharmacological therapy. Below are examples from my own experience, but I am a patient, not a doctor. You should check with your licensed healthcare provider before adopting any of these suggestions.

Nutritional Supplements and Therapies

Nutritional therapy is so important that I devote an entire chapter to it (Chapter 5). Here, I will simply introduce the concept of nutrition and its impact on cancer.

Nutritional therapy is a general term that refers to healing the body by means of diet and vitamin and mineral supplements. Our food is composed of macronutrients and micronutrients. Macronutrients include carbohydrates (sugars and starches), fats, proteins and fiber. Micronutrients are vitamins, minerals and trace elements that cannot be manufactured in the body and so must be consumed. If proper amounts of micronutrients are missing from our diet, then illness results. For example, a vitamin C deficiency can result in scurvy.

Most anti-cancer diets are vegetarian, making use of whole foods which can make a major contribution to health. One of the key aims of a premium diet is to restore digestion with fresh, vital, pure and suitably prepared food.

The use of micronutrient supplements to prevent cancer or to enhance the health of cancer patients is called nutritional therapy and is a hotly debated subject in medical circles. While most medical practitioners do not recommend the taking of vitamin or mineral supplements for cancer patients, there is an increasing number of doctors and health professionals who claim that cancer patients require additional nutrients to augment their immune function. (Many of the long-term cancer survivors with whom I have spoken have taken some kind of nutritional supplement.)

In fact, cancer patients' nutritional needs are greater than the rest of the population. While there is considerable debate over the effectiveness of nutritional supplements, the fact remains that our food sources no longer contain the same levels of vitamins that they had in bygone eras. This is especially the case where the food eaten is not grown organically. The recommended daily amounts of vitamins and minerals are based on minimum standards required in order to prevent illness. They are not based on requirements for optimal body functioning. If you take nutritional supplements, it is essential to have these monitored by a health professional. This is most important because certain cancer cells are enhanced, not retarded, in their function by certain supplements. A number of the books in the Bibliography include practical guidelines on nutrition.

Traditional Chinese Medicine

This is one of the most popular forms of complementary cancer treatment in Australia. Traditional Chinese Medicine (TCM) is a comprehensive system of diagnosis and treatment. The diagnosis is based on a person's history, on observation of the body (especially the tongue), on palpation and on pulse diagnosis. Treatment involves dietary change, acupuncture, medicinal teas, herbs and massage. These various modalities or forms of TCM used for cancer treatment vary according to individual case. Herbs are the most commonly used treatment, followed by acupuncture, Qigong (pronounced 'she gong'), massage, especially acupressure, and even Tai Chi, a gentle form of moving meditation, incorporating breath and movement to help in balancing the body's energy systems. Traditional Chinese medicine requires considerable skill and experience.

Most practitioners of TCM who have been trained in China would acknowledge that their discipline is an adjunctive treatment to conventional Western medicine and that TCM enhances quality of life and alleviates the side-effects of standard treatment, rather than standing on its own.

In contrast to Western medical practice, TCM emphasizes the holistic model of health. Lifestyle, including diet, exercise, thoughts and emotions need to be in a state of balance for vitality and health to be maintained. The Chinese believe that Qi (chi), or vital energy, is an actual physical entity. The 'Qi meridians' are energy fields that are measurable through the pulses, the radial artery, along acupuncture meridians and the tongue. The weakness of certain internal organs can thus be diagnosed. The 'energy meridians' can be stimulated by acupuncture, acupressure, herbs, massage and Qigong. Qigong is a system of body movement, breathing and visualization. Through specific movement, the vital energy of the body, or 'qi force' is cleansed, nurtured and balanced to aid in healing. The Chinese claim that Qigong therapy can aid in such illnesses as cancer, heart disease, arthritis, gynecological problems and most chronic illnesses. The practice of TCM is done with two or more of these modalities working together.

Herbal medicine is the principal mode of TCM. A vast pharmacopoeia of plant, animal and mineral substances make up the Chinese herbal treatments. Herbal medicines tend to be milder than chemical drugs and produce their effects more slowly. One's expectations of them should take this fact into account. The main recommendation as far as TCM is concerned is to seek out a highly experienced practitioner, preferably one who trained in China.

Michael Lerner, in *Choices in Healing* includes a lengthy discussion on the reasons why traditional Chinese medicine is so popular in America. From my own experience and from having spoken to many who have used TCM, Lerner's summary is worth noting for its accuracy:

Traditional Chinese medicine is, in my judgment, one of the most intriguing of the adjunctive therapies for cancer. There is considerable evidence for its benefits in pain management and in alleviating the side-effects of chemotherapy and radiation therapy ... There are also reasons to believe that traditional Chinese medicine may help in the battle to extend life with cancer and to lower the risk of recurrence of cancer.

Herbal Medicine

This incorporates both Eastern and Western use of herbs that are known to build the immune system and have anticancer properties.

There is, as indicated above, a wide range of herbs used in the practice of traditional Chinese medicine. Most of these need to be boiled and drunk in the manner prescribed by the practitioner. There are also a number of herbs that have, for centuries, been known to have immune-boosting and anti-cancer properties. Unfortunately, there are few medical practitioners who have any training or experience with herbal medicine. As stated above, herbal medicines are milder than chemical drugs, so they may take longer to produce effects. However, certain herbs are highly recommended as an adjunct to your mainstream treatment. There are two in particular, which were initially recommended to me by my doctor – a holistic practitioner who has experience with herbal remedies.

The first of these is a Chinese herb called Astragalus. The particular brand I use is Astra 8, a powerful 1:1 liquid extract. Astragalus is a non-toxic herb whose derivatives have been shown to boost immunity, fight cancer and protect against the side effects of chemotherapy. There have been a number of pharmacological studies carried out in recent years suggesting that Astragalus enhances immune function and increases the production of white blood cells, antibodies and interferon. Astragalus also boosts vitality and energy, thus increasing

ts of stress. It is readily available from
or from registered medical herbalists.
pharmacological studies have shown to
iral and immune-boosting properties is an
ɔa called Cat's Claw. This is an amazing
ᴊuᴜᴄᴛᴀnᴄᴇ. when I began to develop flu symptoms last winter, I
dramatically increased my dose of Cat's Claw for 48 hours and
all traces of flu disappeared.

In addition, an herbal tea which is highly recommended for
cleansing the digestive system and for having anti-tumor
properties is green tea, which has in recent years been the subject
of research in Japan. I recommend you consult a herbalist as to
which type of green tea you should buy and the frequency you
should take it. The same applies for ginseng tea, which is
recommended for certain types of cancers.

Oxygen & Ozone Therapies

There has been published scientific data (some going back
over 60 years) that cancer cells do not prosper in a richly
oxygenated (i.e. aerobic) environment. (See for example the
writings of Dr. Otto Warburg.) Ozone is an activated, trivalent
(three atoms) form of oxygen. Oxygen is O2 whereas ozone is
O3. Medical ozone is made when medical grade oxygen is
electrically activated (using an ozone generator) to form ozone.
Ozone is germicidal, bactericidal, and fungicidal.

Three months after my diagnosis, a holistic doctor in Sydney
who practiced integrative medicine (integrating conventional and
complementary treatments) suggested that I try a combination of
ozone therapy and intravenous Vitamin C (30gm twice weekly).
For fifteen months, with regular breaks, I was administered this
therapy. The doctor took out 100 mls of blood from a vein in my
arm. This blood went into a sealed glass bottle, was injected with
ozone from an 'ozonator' machine, and allowed to drip back into
my vein. When that was completed I began the intravenous
vitamin C. I constantly affirmed and believed the benefits of this
treatment. I remain convinced that this combination of

intravenous ozone and vitamin C played an important role in my recovery together with the other lifestyle changes, especially diet, nutritional supplements, meditation, affirmations and prayer.

Pharmacological Therapies

Most pharmacological therapies are in the experimental stage of development. These include shark and bovine cartilage, and Ukrain and Iscador injections. Unconventional pharmacological cancer therapies are not commonly used in America, primarily because few clinical trials have been performed on them. I am including a brief mention of two of them here because of my personal experience with them.

Iscador is a derivative of mistletoe and has long been used as a cancer treatment in Europe. There are numerous references to Iscador in the medical literature that demonstrates its usefulness in cancer. It is available in Germany or Switzerland. Inquire about its use from a holistic medical practitioner.

Another pharmacological cancer treatment was recommended to me by a highly respected cancer surgeon, who claimed that in clinical trials it showed 'much promise.' The treatment is called Ukrain, which is actually half herb – Greater Celandine (Chelidonium majus L.), and half chemotherapy – thiotepa. Celandine, has been used for a very long time in Russian folk medicine. One study demonstrated that when people with cancer were given Ukrain, two measurements of their immune system activity, the levels of circulating lymphocytes and macrophages, rose significantly. This is a sign of the body's increased ability to oppose the spread of cancerous cells. Likewise, clinical trials have demonstrated that Ukrain increases the production of T-helper cells, which help to destroy tumors. At the same time, the measurement of the so-called T-suppressor cells, which hold back the T-helpers and allow tumors to grow, decreased. The clinical notes for physicians indicate that Ukrain is particularly effective for the treatment of breast, bladder, liver, kidney, prostate, ovarian, cervical, small-cell carcinomas and

79

lymphomas. Ukrain is slowly injected intravenously. It is manufactured in Austria. I used it for nearly eighteen months.

CHAPTER SUMMARY

- Make sure that your doctor has experience in treating your particular type of cancer.

- Natural therapists may not be permitted by law to treat cancer. The focus of their work is to enhance your general well being and health and to advise you on diet, nutritional supplements and other adjunctive therapies such as meditation and inner healing. Natural therapies aim at extending quality of life. Remember, though, that quality of life frequently accompanies quantity of life.

- There are a number of different cultures of cancer treatment throughout the world. The philosophical and cultural underpinning of treatment in the U.S., for example, varies considerably from the situation in Europe. American treatments focus on chemotherapy, radiotherapy and surgery.

- Unconventional cancer treatments include some very useful therapies as well as some highly questionable ones. Beware of unscrupulous practitioners who make unsubstantiated claims. Ask for objective evidence of a proposed treatment's success before you agree to pursue a particular treatment. Don't be influenced too much by anecdotal 'evidence.'

- Cancer represents a failure of your healing system. Therefore, do everything possible to improve your overall level of health so that your body's natural defenses can fight the cancer.

- Nutritional therapies have much to offer. While diet alone cannot cure cancer it can certainly assist you in your level of well being and can improve your healing system.

- Traditional Chinese medicine is commonly used as a complementary therapy and has much to offer in helping you to get well again.

- Herbal medicine can greatly help to boost your immune function.

- Pharmacological therapies – especially such treatments as Ukrain show much promise – although they are still in the experimental stage of development.

ജ 5 ര

NUTRITION AND DIET

AFTER MY DIAGNOSIS, I LISTENED TO CLAIMS AND COUNTERCLAIMS ABOUT DIET AND NUTRITIONAL THERAPIES, ESPECIALLY VITAMIN, MINERAL AND HERBAL SUPPLEMENTS. Who was I to believe? The answer at the time seemed to be that a highly nutritious diet, combined with certain vitamin supplements to assist in maintaining stamina, could only help.

Nutrition and diet, like most of the topics in this book, are subjects that involve choices about the way in which we live – these are lifestyle choices. Some cancer patients decide to stay with the diets they had before the onset of their illness, and there are those who claim that certain extremely rigorous dietary manipulations (such as the Gerson Diet, the Bruess Diet and a strict macrobiotic diet) have cured their cancers.

The main aim of this chapter is to give you clear guidelines that I found useful on my healing path and to clarify the confusing array of information that is out there on diet and nutrition. I recognize that every cancer patient's nutritional needs vary, so these are only guidelines, not prescriptive statements about what you should be eating or supplements you should be taking. This information is a combination of professional advice given to me and intensive reading on the subject.

Most health professionals who espouse a holistic philosophy (that is, they look at the person, not just his/her symptoms) believe that it is not merely a 'good' or a 'bad' diet that is the chief determinant of a person's level of health. Factors such as emotional and mental health also exert important influences on whether or not we stay well. At times the body's self-regulating mechanisms compensate for people's poor nutrition and they stay remarkably healthy. Their apparent good health, in spite of poor, unbalanced diets may be explained because they lead balanced lives. They are happy people who enjoy peace of mind. We need to be comfortable with our diets and know that they are assisting our healing. Only then can adherence to wholesome, anti-cancer diets help in maintaining our wellness and assist us in our recoveries.

There is plenty of nutritional evidence that diet is one of the key factors that stimulate and activate the body's own healing activity. If food is the body's 'fuel' then it is self-evident that if we supply our bodies with 'premium' fuel they will function better, including their immune systems. However, there is not much to be gained by adopting a strict anti-cancer diet grudgingly because it is not likely to be of great benefit. Being in a depressed state tends to lower immune function.

A person who has a strong and positive outlook on life will want to embrace a nutritional regime that will optimize her chances of recovery. Current medical opinion is that a poor, unbalanced diet is a contributing cause of certain cancers. The analogy that your body's performance is, to a large extent, determined by the quality of fuel it runs on, is all the more applicable when your body is being stressed by toxic treatments such as chemotherapy. At such a time your body certainly needs 'premium octane fuel' to maintain, if not enhance, its performance.

A QUESTION OF CHOICE

There are a number of ways to approach the question of anti-cancer diets. The most obvious of these is to recognize that each cancer patient's situation and needs are different and that each person will respond differently to diet and nutritional therapy. Furthermore, diet and nutritional therapy must be viewed in the overall context of other lifestyle modifications, especially meditation, positive thinking and peer support. Diet is only one aspect, albeit a vital one, of a total approach to healing.

The key dietary choices are as follows:

- Stay with the diet you were on before being diagnosed.

- Adopt a 'maintenance' (or long-term) healthy whole foods diet which is low in calories and proteins and which replaces animal protein foods with fish and soy foods. Such a diet avoids substances known to be harmful to health. For those whose diets have been unbalanced and lacking in nutrition before their diagnoses, a dietary change such as this can make an important contribution to their health.

- Adopt an individualized, and in some cases, an intensive nutritional program such as the Gerson Diet, the Bruess diet, the Gawler diet (as set out in his book *You Can Conquer Cancer*), or a macrobiotic diet (see Glossary). Many people have experienced dramatic improvements in their health by following such diets. This is because these diets cleanse the body of accumulated toxins and contribute to the more efficient functioning of the vital organs. There are some who have claimed that such a diet has (in conjunction with other therapies, such as vitamin and mineral supplements) cured them of their cancers. This has also been the case with specialized nutritional regimes such as the grape juice diet and the Breuss Diet.

There are a number of basic principles for nutritional cancer therapy upon which most nutritionists and holistic doctors would agree. These include:

- The body should be detoxified.

- Any vitamin and mineral imbalances need to be corrected.

- Digestion needs to be restored and the diet should consist of only fresh, vital, pure and suitably prepared food.

- You need to have a positive attitude, both in general and to your diet in particular.

When you affirm and fully believe that your diet, in conjunction with everything else that you are doing, is helping you to get well again, your mind is sending strong 'live' messages to your body. In time, your body will respond.

It is a pity that the concept of 'detoxification' is most commonly associated with 'alternative' medicine, especially because conventional medicine widely acknowledges the toxic and carcinogenic impact made on our bodies by many substances in our environment, not the least of these being cigarettes. For centuries, fasting has been acknowledged as a means of removing impurities and cleansing the body. Changing to a healthy whole foods diet can have much the same effect, although more gradually than other forms of detoxification. Years of eating processed food with chemical additives will do little to strengthen the immune system and help the body resist the onset or effects of illness.

Vitamin and mineral supplementation and the role of juicing fresh vegetables (particularly carrots) are discussed below. From the time of my diagnosis, my medical advice (including from a leading surgeon) suggested that all cancer patients require vitamin and mineral supplements, although this needs to be carefully tailored to each person.

OPTIONS FOR NUTRITIONAL THERAPIES

The following options for nutritional therapies are a synthesis of what the experts in this field advise:

- Rely on natural sources, namely, whole food and juices. This is a preferred option.

- Follow the recommendations of a health professional about taking vitamin, mineral and, perhaps, amino acid supplements each day. This may include an intensive regime of supplements, especially to compensate for the lowering of the immune system when undergoing radical treatments such as chemotherapy or radiation. (At the end of this chapter, there is a recommended list of supplements for those undergoing such treatments.)

- Vitamin C supplementation, either 8-10 grams daily or to bowel tolerance. (Excessive vitamin C can cause a loose bowel so you need to find the right dosage to suit you.) The benefits of vitamin C have been extensively researched over many years. There is some evidence that very high doses of vitamin C given intravenously inhibit tumor growth.

WHAT MAKES A HEALING DIET

The basic 'rule' of a healing diet is that it is a natural, whole food diet. In other words, it concentrates on the basic food groups of fruit, vegetables and grains with a deliberate avoidance of refined and processed foods. Refined foods are such things as white flour, sugar, cakes, ice cream, chocolate and soft drinks. Processed foods include the majority of meats sold in delicatessens and most fast and takeaway foods. Unless it is organic, most of the chicken and meat we buy contains antibiotics, pesticides and other chemicals. Some chemical food additives can be harmful and lead to chemical sensitivities and allergy problems. Refined and processed foods might provide energy but have reduced vitamin and mineral content compared to whole foods. Refined foods also tend to be high in saturated fats, which can be harmful.

Nutrition books frequently tell us to cut down on our calories. It is a truism that most of us tend to over eat, rather than under eat. A number of researchers on the connection between diet and cancer, including Professor Ray Kearney, of the University of Sydney, claim there is evidence that under-eating has benefits for the body's self-healing capacity. The calorie restriction he recommends is achieved by limiting food intake to specific meal times – no 'grazing.'

Fat

Eating too much of the wrong kinds of fats can impair the body's ability to heal. Fats are classified into saturated, monounsaturated and poly-unsaturated. Two of the poly-unsaturated fats, omega 3 and omega 6 are essential nutrients. In other words, the body cannot manufacture them and they must come from the diet. Nutrients such as cholesterol are non-essential, because the body can make them from other nutrients. If the ratio of the omega 3's and the omega 6's is badly out of balance (as with the high-fat, high-meat Western diet) this may ultimately lead to chronic illness such as cancer. A brief but highly informative discussion on the fats–cancer connection is found in Section Seven, Chapter 80 of *Fats that Heal, Fats that Kill*, by Udo Erasmus. The essence of Erasmus's argument is that saturated fatty acids (such as those found in fried foods) interfere with oxygen use in our cells. Heat, hydrogenation, light and oxygen produce chemically altered fat products that are toxic to our cells. These fats may play a significant part in bringing about the onset of cancer. The recommendation for a healing diet for all cancer patients as far as fats are concerned include:

- Reduce your fat intake by eliminating deep-fried foods.

- Substitute soy products and goat's milk or goat's milk products for cow's milk products. Try cottage cheese and yoghurt. Avoid margarine and vegetable shortenings as they contain harmful substances called trans-fatty acids.

- Reduce or eliminate meat and unskinned poultry. (The issue of a vegetarian diet is discussed below.)

- Eliminate polyunsaturated vegetable oils from your diet by avoiding safflower, sunflower, corn, soy, peanut and cottonseed oils. These oils, unlike olive oil, are unstable when heated and cancer patients must avoid rancid products.

- Sauté in water, rather than fry. If frying use extra virgin olive oil.

- Increase consumption of omega 3 fatty acids by eating deep sea fish and/or flaxseed oil or meal regularly.

Protein

We mostly rely on animal foods for protein: meat, poultry, fish, milk and milk products. Begin to replace animal protein in the diet with fish and soy protein or at least buy organic meat and chicken. Either way, cut down on animal protein, as it contains saturated fat that places stress on the digestive system. Remember that meat is a major source of saturated fat in the diet. It also contains (unless it is organic) many environmental toxins, such as chemicals used in commercial farming. Chicken presents the same toxic hazards as the meat of cows, sheep and pigs and may contain even more added hormones, as well as salmonella bacteria (if it is not cooked well).

Vegetable sources of protein are beans, grains and some nuts. Design some of your meals around carbohydrates and vegetables: stir-fries with rice, or pasta and vegetables, or salads and bread. Cutting down on protein will free up energy, put less strain on your liver and kidneys and allow your immune system to function more efficiently.

Grains and beans contain carbohydrate and fiber as well as protein, so you can eat more of them without having an excess of protein. Limit your intake of nuts mainly to raw almonds and raw cashews (in moderation because they also contain quite a high fat content). Soybeans and tofu products are also a useful protein source.

Fruit and Vegetables

These should be eaten plentifully, preferably of the organic variety, if they're available, or if your budget will allow. Besides supplying you with essential vitamins and minerals, fruit and vegetables will provide the fiber that is so important for your digestive system.

A Vegetarian Diet?

I have posed this question because there are very different opinions as to whether a vegetarian diet impedes the development of cancer or, indeed, whether it will help to improve and restore health if you already have cancer.

Not so many years ago, vegetarian diets were followed mainly by those with a particular religious or ethical belief. Things have changed and these days a sizeable number of people choose to be vegetarian for a variety of other reasons. That is not to say that all vegetarian diets are healthy, as some may still contain significant amounts of sugar and fat. A vegetarian diet needs to be monitored to avoid protein or other deficiencies. There needs to be a variety of grains, such as corn, rice, wheat, and legumes (such as beans and lentils). Shortly after my diagnosis when I changed to a vegetarian diet, I followed my doctor's strong recommendation that I modify it by eating deep sea fish such as blue-eyed cod or salmon twice a week to increase my intake of omega 3 essential fatty acids.

For a cancer patient to make a dietary change makes as much sense as smokers who are diagnosed with lung cancer or heart disease to stop smoking. Research has established that vegetarian diets lower levels of known carcinogens such as saturated fats and excess protein. Therefore such a diet may help to alter the way tumor cells process fat and thereby prevent, or at least slow, the runaway growth that characterizes fatal cancers. The evidence linking the high intake of fat, protein and sugar to colon, prostate and breast cancer in later life is starting to accumulate. So again, you should seriously consider the benefits of a vegetarian diet, or at least a predominantly vegetarian diet.

Thousands of cancer patients follow a whole food dietary regime, or a variation of it – one of the anti-cancer diets that are so similar to a low-fat diet followed by people with a heart condition. Dietary considerations are one of the basic tools for getting well.

Juicing

Vegetable juicing is a valuable supplement to a healing diet. While juicing vegetables is the best source of nutrients to build and regenerate our bodies, eating fruit is the best way to cleanse them. Vegetable juices such as carrot, celery and beetroot are full of enzymes, vitamins, minerals and trace elements that are much more easily assimilated than solid food. The fresh, 'living' nutrients in juices (when the fiber is removed) can get into the bloodstream and to the cellular level in minutes, without the time consuming and energy-depleting process of digestion. They are palatable (green juices slightly less so) and help restore energy levels. They are particularly valuable as an adjunct to chemotherapy or radiotherapy. Juices should always be freshly prepared because when they are stored they readily oxidize, thus losing their nutritional benefit. My preferred juicer is one that separates the pulp from the juice and, importantly, retains the enzymes. Most health food stores stock appropriate juicers.

As well as the above-mentioned vegetable juices, I have found the juice of young barley, which is marketed under various brand names such as Green Barley Plus, Barley Green or Green Magma, a very useful aid in healing. It is another valuable source of 'living' nutrients and is a concentrated food of proteins, vitamins, enzymes, minerals, and, most importantly, chlorophyll, which cleanses and oxygenates the blood. Enzymes have a critical function in the body. They are the catalysts for all chemical changes, including the digestion of food, sending oxygen from our lungs to our blood and cells and synthesizing proteins from amino acids to make muscle. There is some evidence from research in Japan to indicate that barley green helps inhibit cancer cells. Unlike many synthetically produced vitamins, barley green is much more readily absorbed and assimilated. I take a glass of barley green (with 20 ml of aloe vera juice and 20 ml of chlorophyll) first thing each morning and again an hour before the evening meal. I also have a large glass of carrot and celery juice mid-morning and mid-afternoon. I have read numerous testimonials from people who claim to have cured various chronic illnesses, including cancer, from barley green and vegetable juices.

The Gerson Therapy

This therapy is based upon the work of Dr. Max Gerson, a German physician who, after the coming to power of the Nazis in the 1930's, emigrated to the United States for a number of decades. Gerson believed that cancer results from an impaired immune system. He believed that a healthy body would react to, and eliminate cancer. Of all the alternative nutritional cancer therapies, Gerson's has been subjected to more clinical trials and investigations than any other. This is a diet and detoxification program consisting of a combination of juices, vegetables, coffee enemas and enzymes. Of the dozens of patients I have talked to, few have actually used this therapy. This is so partially because its most experienced practitioners are at the Gerson Institute in Tijuana, Mexico and partially because this is a difficult and demanding regime, requiring a great deal of dedication, perseverance and faith. Because this is a rigorous treatment it should be undertaken only with a doctor's supervision. A list of doctors conversant with this treatment can be obtained from the Internet.

Micronutrients – Which Vitamins Should I Take?

This is one of those near impossible questions to answer because each person's nutritional needs are different. This is not the place for a detailed discussion of each of the main vitamin and mineral supplements, nor of some of the main herbs used by herbalists to complement cancer treatment. It is significant, however, that every long-term cancer survivor with whom I have spoken takes some form of vitamin, mineral or herbal supplement. It is also worth noting that the majority of conventional medical practitioners do not endorse the taking of supplements, mainly because this is an area with which they are unfamiliar. They believe that with a nutritious diet supplements are unnecessary. In theory, they are right. In practice, this is not the case. Firstly, much fresh produce has been in cold storage and has therefore lost a good deal of its nutritional value; secondly, cancer patients have an increased nutritional demand because their immune systems are under greater stress and because of the toxic treatments they may be receiving.

The following list of nutritional supplements represents a general guideline only. It is essential that you have your supplements monitored by a licensed health practitioner – such as a medical doctor (MD), naturopathic doctor (one who is trained in nutrition, an ND), or a herbalist.

- Vitamins A (4000 iu and D "natural nutrition" two daily (divided dose)
- Vitamin C (preferably non-acidic calcium ascorbate containing bioflavanoids) 8,000-10,000 mg daily (3 teaspoons per day)
- Vitamin E (400–500iu) twice daily
- Vitamin B complex one 500 mg tablet daily
- Folic acid one 500 mcg tablet daily
- Selenium (sodium selenite drops or SuperSelenium drops) twice daily **Caution:** selenium is toxic in doses of 5 mg per kg body weight in an acute form and can cause a variety of effects from garlic breath to liver damage and birth defects.

Men need more than women as sperm contains high levels of selenium.

- Flaxseed oil (refrigerated only) two teaspoons daily
- Melatonin (a hormone, not a vitamin) one tablet at bedtime. **Caution:** There are recommendations against melatonin for those with leukemia, lymphoma and auto-immune diseases. Not recommended in pregnancy or those under the age of 35. It is reported to have anti-cancer effects for breast and prostate cancer.
- Coenzyme Q10 30mg twice daily

There are some holistic medical practitioners who recommend intravenous Vitamin C, especially during chemotherapy or radiation therapy. Discuss this possibility with your doctor. I found it helpful in the first year after I was diagnosed. My daily vitamin and mineral intake included the above list. I realize that for some people this may be financially prohibitive. If that is the case, then my advice, based on medical advice given to me is that you consider taking Vitamins A, C and E. These are powerful antioxidants and assist the body to detoxify and therefore better able to deal with fighting the cancer.

HERBAL IMMUNE STIMULANTS

I had the rare and good fortune to have a doctor who was also a medical herbalist. It was on this basis that he recommended I take the following herbal supplements. Cat's Claw (botanical name: Uncaria Tomentosa) and Astragalus, a Chinese herb that helps build white blood cells and is a powerful blood purifier.

I took Cat's claw liquid, one teaspoon twice daily. It is documented to have strong anti-cancer properties. I took 'Astragalus 8' or 'Astraforte' (from health food stores) one teaspoon twice daily.

SOME CONSIDERATIONS DURING CHEMOTHERAPY/RADIOTHERAPY

Although I did not take chemotherapy or radiation therapy, if you decide to you should consider taking certain supplements to help your immune system recover from these powerful treatments.

Chemotherapy consists of treatment by cytotoxic drugs – drugs designed to kill cells. Chemotherapy kills both healthy cells and tumor cells and can either be used in a localized region of the body, at the site of the cancer, or more generally (systemically) where the cancer has metastasized or spread to other organs or areas of the body.

The purpose of chemotherapy is to shrink the tumors, to control the growth of the cancer, or to eradicate it altogether. Sometimes chemotherapy and/or radiotherapy is used as an adjunctive, or secondary treatment, to surgery. These treatments are also designed to alleviate symptoms and to prolong life.

The side effects of these treatments depend to a very considerable degree on the type and the dosage of the chemotherapy or radiotherapy. Some people do not experience any side effects, others have only minimal reactions. Side effects may include nausea, vomiting and hair loss. Usually such reactions quickly disappear when the treatment is stopped. Also, remember that each individual reacts differently. It is not fair to generalize. However, the fact remains that both these treatments are toxic. This is a situation that warrants taking vitamin and mineral supplements to counteract any adverse effects. Here are a few suggestions.

NUTRITIONAL SUGGESTIONS

There are an ever-increasing number of doctors who are recognizing the need for vitamin and mineral supplementation, particularly at a time of chronic illness. *As previously mentioned, such supplementation should be supervised and monitored by a*

94

medical professional. The following recommendations have been compiled by a nutritionist.

- Vitamin A: Useful for healing damaged tissue.
- Vitamin C: Has an anti-viral effect and provides a general physical boost. (Best to use non-acidic vitamin C.)
- Vitamin E: Oxygenation of the cells; cell repair and healing.
- Flaxseed Oil: Dispense sticky blood and platelet aggregation.
- Vitamin B Complex: Anti-stress formula.
- Vitamin B12: Preferably by injection.
- Biostrath: A Swiss preparation restoring appetite, immunity and radiation protection.
- Acidophilus Powder: To restore the correct bacteria in the bowel which chemotherapy or radiation can upset.
- Make sure you have a high fluid intake and that it is pure, filtered water.
- Drink four or more juices (carrot, carrot and beetroot, barley green) a day. They are rich in essential enzymes and help to oxygenate the blood. Avoid this if you have a problem with diabetes, as the natural sugar in the juices may be a problem.
- Drink dandelion coffee rather than caffeine.
- Drink herbal teas rather than ordinary tea.
- Wholemeal pastas, for example, soba (made from buckwheat) and other grain pastas.
- No added sugar jams.
- The following beverages are good to drink while undergoing treatment: Lloyd's biodynamic grape juice; Eden Biodynamic vegetable juices; Biotta vegetable juices. All are available from good health food stores.

POSITIVE ATTITUDE TOWARDS FOOD

Most health professionals would agree that the most important thing you need as a cancer patient is a positive attitude. This applies to food as to all of life. You need to believe firmly that the course of your disease can be favorably

95

influenced by eating wholesome, nutritious food that will enhance your metabolic function. Don't be put off by lack of encouragement in this area. In the early days after my diagnosis my oncologist told me not to punish myself with rigorous diets that will make absolutely no difference in the course of my cancer. I chose to ignore that advice in the light of the stories of people who had made remarkable recoveries from their illnesses. All of them spoke of the importance of diet in maintaining their wellness. Sure, diet, of itself, cannot possibly cure cancer but diet and nutritional supplements can certainly help your body to fight it. Don't listen to negative talk on this subject. Embrace your diet in a positive frame of mind. Any dietary change will take some time to adapt to but do not be deterred. Also remember that occasional 'lapses' will do you no harm. It is more important to be happy about what you eat.

CHAPTER SUMMARY

- Diet and nutrition play an important role in activating the body's healing activity.

- Cancer patients require premium nutrition if they are to enhance their chance of recovery.

- The main principle underlying any 'anti-cancer' diet is that the body needs to be detoxified, and that vitamin and mineral imbalances need to be corrected.

- Your food should be primarily a healthy whole food diet that concentrates on the basic food groups of fruit, vegetables and grains, and avoids refined and processed foods containing white flour, sugar, cakes and ice-cream.

- Having a positive attitude towards food is very important. You should feel good about the dietary choices you make and realize that your nutrition contributes significantly to your healing.

ಖ 6 ಆ

LIVING WITH CANCER

THIS CHAPTER EXPLORES SOME OF THE PHYSICAL, PSYCHOLOGICAL AND EMOTIONAL ISSUES RELATING TO A CANCER DIAGNOSIS. The topics discussed include:

- Problems of living with cancer
- Cancer as a turning point
- Stress management
- Meditation – the silent healer
- Pain control
- Keeping a journal
- Keeping your life in balance
- Humor
- Spirituality

PROBLEMS ENCOUNTERED
WHEN LIVING WITH CANCER

As I discussed at the beginning of this book, each cancer patient has a unique set of variables in the same way that each of us has a unique personality, genes and so on. Therefore, I run the risk of generalizing when discussing the problems of living with cancer.

The issues discussed in this chapter relate to the problems concerned with the treatment of this illness and those that relate to lifestyle. Some of these matters have also been touched in other chapters. This is unavoidable.

The first set of problems relates to the initial response to the diagnosis. These are issues such as choice of a doctor with whom you feel comfortable, choice of treatment, coping with the trauma of treatment and living with a progressive illness. The second sets of issues are broader matters pertaining to 'lifestyle.'

Psychological research in the United States and United Kingdom has shown unresolved emotional issues frequently occur as causative factors in a cancer diagnosis. Research has established a reasonable correlation between the suppression of emotional trauma and the onset of the disease. This was also a finding of Dr. Ainslie Meares, who noted that an unusually large number of his cancer patients had experienced a trauma such as divorce, bereavement or job loss in the eighteen-month to two year period prior to diagnosis. These patients had often carried a high degree of stress with them – stress brought on partly through suppressing feelings of guilt, resentment, powerlessness and hopelessness, as well as having the inability to express their emotions. Such patients tended to be introverted and tended to have low self-esteem.

A cancer diagnosis can exacerbate such problems in a person's life – even more so if the diagnosis is unexpected. A patient can feel isolated, especially if his routine has been severely interrupted. There may be loss of income, subsequently putting a strain on finances. Family relationships may be strained and one's life can very easily be pushed out of balance. These are some of the problems. What, then, are the solutions? Well, the good news from speaking to survivors and reading their testimonies, is that one of the common threads to their stories is that cancer has proved a painful, daunting, yet challenging experience through which they have emerged the richer. Richer in what way? Ironic as this may sound, cancer has brought inner healing in their lives. It has brought about a greater self-awareness. They gained self awareness in terms of compassion, love, creativity by means of positive thinking, and a recognition that spirituality is an integral part of life. Commonly, cancer patients have reported that their illness has, strangely, brought them peace of mind. Exactly how this was achieved is the main theme of this chapter.

CANCER AS A TURNING POINT

In 1989, Dr. Lawrence Le Shan, a psychologist and one of the pioneers of psychological interventions for cancer wrote a book called *Cancer as a Turning Point*. His research had shown him that a considerable proportion of cancer patients exhibit a sense of hopelessness. This hopelessness in the face of past emotional experiences duly affected immune function and left the person vulnerable to a chronic illness such as cancer. Le Shan argued that cancer can be regarded as a 'turning point' – the need to re-evaluate what is important and what is unimportant in life. For some patients this reassessment happens spontaneously; for others, it comes as a gradual shift in consciousness.

In my case, this shift in consciousness happened quite dramatically. My cancer was discovered accidentally during a routine umbilical hernia operation. I hadn't for a moment expected to be told that I had widespread cancer throughout my abdomen and that there was not very much that could be done for me medically. Yet, even in the turmoil of emotions that were part of the shock that had set in, I realized with crystal clarity that my life was out of balance and had been for several years. I had been searching for another job for quite a while and had all but given up, knowing that age had caught up with me. I had become somewhat bitter about a number of things and I harbored deep-seated resentments that I seemed powerless to change. In addition, I was always worried about the past or the future and I was certainly not enjoying the present. People told me that I was a highly stressed person. Indeed, one person had repeatedly warned me that if I did not learn to get my stress under control that I would end up with cancer due to adrenal exhaustion! As I lay in that hospital bed immediately after surgery, those words echoed in my ears.

I recognize now that it was not so much my behavior and attitudes that were to 'blame' for my cancer. Rather, I interpreted my cancer as the product of past emotional experiences that in turn led to beliefs and behaviors that over a long period of time, were detrimental to my health by weakening my immune system. Within a day of receiving the bad news I made a commitment to turn my life around, to beat this cancer and not to accept this doctor's grim prognosis. My entire consciousness had shifted. I am not for a moment suggesting that initially (and for many months afterwards) I was free from the clutches of fear. Far from it – fear ebbed and flowed depending on what the test results showed. Gradually, however, helped along by others, I learned to control and master this fear.

As the weeks turned into months I began to feel that I had passed through the eye of the storm and that life, cancer not withstanding, was in certain respects better than it had been before. To have been so brazenly confronted with my mortality had challenged me to survive. At the same time it had also produced an entirely new perspective on living. In summary, it had taught me that life was very precious and sacred and that I should treasure it. My cancer diagnosis was, as it were, a dramatic catalyst of change. I recognize, of course, that each individual's response is different. From my own experience and from observing others with this illness, it seems to me that in order to survive we not only need to seek out the best that conventional and complementary treatments have to offer, but also we need to adopt a positive mind-set.

The technique for helping to achieve this is the subject of the remainder of this chapter – but first, an inspirational verse.

The longer I live, the more I realize the impact of attitudes on life. Attitude to me is more important than the past, than education, than money, than successes, than what other people think or say or do. It is more important than appearance, giftedness or skill. It will make or break a company ... a church ... a home. The remarkable thing is that you have a choice every day regarding the attitude you will embrace for that day. We cannot change the inevitable ... the only thing we can do is play on the one string we have, and that is our attitude. I am convinced that life is 10 percent what happens to me and 90 per cent how I react to it. And so it is with you ... You are in charge of your attitude.

—AUTHOR UNKNOWN.

STRESS MANAGEMENT: CALMING MENTAL, EMOTIONAL AND NERVOUS ANXIETY

In his book *Choices in Healing* Michael Lerner makes the point that probably the most common problems facing the cancer patient revolve around relationships. That is not to suggest, of course, that relationship problems are unique to cancer patients. However, they have a poignancy to cancer sufferers. A number of books deal extensively with this subject. One of these is *Why People Don't Heal – And How They Can*, by Carolyn Myss. The question of how relationships can be related to a cancer diagnosis is far beyond the scope of this discussion. It is, however, important to recognize that a range of relationship issues – things such as negative childhood experiences (for example, sexual or psychological abuse), a failed marriage, friends who distance themselves from you upon hearing of your cancer, can all, in their own ways, contribute to harming or healing you. In Lerner's words, "An experience like cancer tends to mobilize both the supportive and the negative potential in the social networks that surround each of us."

One of the truisms of a cancer diagnosis is that it strips away all falseness; it reveals the truth about your own life and about the lives of those who surround you. A great challenge of a cancer diagnosis is that it provides the opportunity to heal relationships – and in some cases to explore and to come to terms with yourself; with unresolved emotional issues which have the potential to block your healing. The illness itself can be a turning point that gives you permission for the first time to explore being yourself.

As I indicated in the opening chapter, one of the chief causes of the stress that comes with a cancer diagnosis is fear: fear of being confronted with your mortality, fear of the treatment and its side-effects, fear of the treatment not working, fear of losing your job (and in some cases your livelihood) and fear of the effect of this diagnosis on your family. Fear, in one form or another, is a universal problem that comes with a cancer diagnosis. We really need to address that fear. On a mental level, knowledge dispels fear, while on an emotional level love is the greatest antidote.

The 'trick' is to learn to be able to let go of your fears so that at an emotional level and, hopefully, in turn, on a physical level, you can begin your healing journey. Only by learning to let go of your fear will you achieve peace of mind, which is a precondition of healing. This is all well and good, but how do we begin this journey? At a practical level, what do we actually do to combat mental, emotional and nervous anxiety? There are simple things that we can do to help cope with the stressful situation of a cancer diagnosis. The first of these are breathing exercises, which are helpful when practiced regularly, to encourage relaxation. You may start with only five to ten minutes for each exercise and slowly build up to a longer period.

Exercise 1: Counting the breath

Sit comfortably with your back straight and your hands facing upward resting on your lap. Be still for a few moments and become aware of your body posture. Slowly close your eyes. Take a few deep breaths. With each in-breath, imagine that you are breathing in peace and love; and each out-breath breathes out any tension.

Now, breathing naturally, count your breaths on either the exhalation or inhalation from one to ten, repeating the procedure two or three times. When thoughts arise, as inevitably they will, simply allow them to come and go, keeping your attention focused on counting the breaths. If your attention wanders and you lose count, gently bring back your attention to your breathing and start counting from one again.

Exercise 2: Observing the breath

Sit comfortably with a straight back, as in Exercise 1. Focus your attention on your breathing without trying to influence it in any way. Follow the rhythm of your breathing cycle and notice the point where your breath changes from inhale to exhale. Do this for a few minutes. Merely observe what is going on with your breathing cycle. At the end of a few minutes bring your awareness back to your body. Then, when you are ready, slowly open your eyes. Experience the feeling of relaxation.

Exercise 3: Focusing

Start as with the previous two exercises. Then, breathing naturally, focus your attention on the sensation at the tip of your nostrils as the breath flows in and out of your body. Again, keep a passive attitude to the thoughts and images that pass through your mind and, if your attention wanders, gently bring it back to the task in hand. After a few minutes you may like to switch your concentration to the movement of your abdomen as you inhale and exhale. A further variation of this technique is to focus your attention on the space between breaths – the moment of complete stillness. Again, if your mind wanders, gently bring it back to your breathing.

Exercise 4: Mindfulness

Sit comfortably, in the same manner as in the previous exercises. Read and learn the following sequence by repeating each phrase in your mind. As you turn your attention to that part of your body indicated, feel a change taking place; feel tension being released. As you come to the end of the exercise feel a harmonizing of body and mind. Focus your awareness on experiencing a sense of peace and calm. Remember that none of these relaxation exercises involves thinking; they are entirely experiential. The relaxed state you are aiming for is not intended to put you to sleep (although that may occasionally happen if you're feeling tired). Rather, these exercises are designed to bring peace, calm and an 'inner awareness' to your everyday living. The sequence is as follows:

I relax the muscles at the top of my head.
I relax the muscles in my face and head.
I am beginning to relax.
I am relaxing the muscles in my neck.
I am relaxing the muscles of my shoulders.
I am beginning to feel calm and relaxed.
I am relaxing the muscles in my back.
I am relaxing the muscles in my abdomen.
I am becoming calmer and more relaxed all the time.
I am relaxing the muscles of my legs and feet.
I am relaxing the muscles of my arms and hands.
I am becoming calmer and more relaxed all the time.
My body is calm. I feel perfectly calm. I feel at peace.

Try these four exercises and practice them regularly. Only by regular practice will you gain a benefit from them. The deep relaxation these exercises help to promote prepares the way for healing at all levels.

It is important to put aside a regular time each day to practice being still. Why should this be so? Simply because it is only by being still that we are able to experience what one writer has called 'oneness,' a time when we can reconnect with the body, let go of fear and anxiety and just be focused on the present moment. After all, the present moment is all that we actually have. The above exercises help us focus on inner stillness. Even if they bring only temporary peace of mind, they have achieved an important goal in helping you to heal, or at least enhance, your emotional well being.

HINTS TO ALLEVIATE STRESS

- EXERCISE REGULARLY. This need not be vigorous. Going for a walk, or doing fifteen minutes of Tai Chi or yoga each morning can be a very good start to the day. Make sure that you do some form of exercise at least twice each day.

- TRY TO AVOID ALCOHOL, SEDATIVES AND ANTIHISTAMINES as these can depress both your system and your emotions.

- A HERBAL TREATMENT THAT IS USEFUL FOR ANXIETY IS VALERIAN. This is available in tablet or liquid (tincture) form. The latter is more effective. Ten drops in a little warm water can be very useful for calming during the day.

- A HERBAL TREATMENT FOR DEPRESSION IS ST JOHN'S WORT (HYPERICUM). Contrary to recent sensationalist media reports, St John's Wort is non-toxic. It is also available in tablet or liquid form – the latter being faster acting. Both Valerian and St John's Wort are available from most health food stores and pharmacies.

- FOR TIMES OF STRESS AND ANXIETY, AND TO SOOTHE JANGLED NERVES, BACH FLOWER RESCUE REMEDY, A HOMOEOPATHIC SOLUTION, REALLY WORKS. It is also available from health food stores and selected pharmacies.

- HAVE WHAT DR. BERNIE SIEGEL CALLS 'HEALING MOMENTS' EACH DAY. By this he means moments when you make time for stillness. Such moments might include a prayer, patting a dog or a cat, a few moments of contemplation, looking at a beautiful scene or even cultivating stillness through observing your breath. These 'healing moments' de-stress at a spiritual level.

- WHEN STRESSFUL EVENTS OR THOUGHTS OCCUR (SUCH AS BAD NEWS IN THE FORM OF A TEST RESULT), TAKE TIME FOR A 'HEALING MOMENT' in which you either say a prayer to hand over your burden to God, or make a positive affirmation such as 'I am grateful for the blessings I receive daily,' or 'Each day my body is healing itself,' or 'Every day and in every way I am getting better and better.'

- AS ALREADY STATED IN CHAPTER 2, THE POWER OF BELIEF IS VERY GREAT. Saying affirmations aloud takes them into the realm of the subconscious. Always program your mind to the positive (all the more when things are not going too well). Affirmations are not an exercise in self-delusion. They are designed to cancel out a programmed negative thought. They can really help to turn the corner mentally and, in time, physically as well.

MEDITATION – THE SILENT HEALER

As an aid to recovering from a major illness such as cancer, meditation has been shown to be a powerful silent healer. Dr. Ainslie Meares from Melbourne, Australia was a pioneer in promoting the health-giving possibilities of meditation. Since the early 1980's, Dr. Ian Gawler's work in Australia with cancer support groups and his 'wellness' residential courses for people affected by cancer have centered on meditation as a tool to assist in improving patients' quality of life as well as to assist in the recovery process.

The regular practice of meditation is an extremely useful remedy for stress and for bringing the body into a state of deep relaxation. When the body is relaxed its capacity for self-healing is enhanced. What then is meditation? It has many definitions. The common thread is that meditation involves an altered or pure state of consciousness. No, there is nothing mystical or 'New Age' about it. In his book *Spontaneous Healing*, Dr. Andrew Weil makes a simple but comprehensive statement about what meditation is when he writes that meditation is a technique to break the addiction of thought; in essence, it is directed concentration.

We all know that throughout our waking hours our minds are constantly bombarded with thoughts. They change from one subject to another in a rapidly flowing stream of consciousness. By meditating we enter a state of pure consciousness that is free of thoughts. It is not 'emptying the mind' rather it is stilling the mind and allowing us to live in the present moment. This allows us to let go of the past and the future, which is what preoccupies most of our thoughts, and, at least for a short time, stay in the moment. The breathing exercises above are simple forms of meditation whose aim is to let go of any stress and anxiety by this relaxation response.

Meditation is, therefore, both a state and an activity – the art of stilling, or letting go, of the mind. In doing this, we are moving into a deeply relaxed state and giving the body a chance to utilize its self-healing capacities to the maximum. Meditation is also all about mindfulness, or being focused on the present moment. In his book *Spontaneous Healing*, Dr. Weil makes the point that meditation is both simple and difficult. Simple because the method is nothing more than maintaining focused attention; difficult because it requires us to harness the mind from its constant habit of darting from one thought to another.

Most cancer support groups spend a short time in group meditation. It is an excellent way to be introduced to this simple, gentle, healing art. Also, the support of the group is a strong encourager to keep up with your practice. This is an important benefit of joining such a group.

Visualization is one particular form of meditating that is often used as an aid in recovery from cancer. One of the pioneers of this technique was Dr. Carl Simonton and his wife Stephanie, whose book *Getting Well Again* has become a classic in its field. In it they describe how the mind can be trained, through positive attitudes, relaxation, visualization and in other ways, to battle cancer.

Visualization is all about using mind–body communication to reinforce positive images of recovery. The way this is done is by connecting the mind to the will through the visual cortex of the brain. The mental imagery process occurs by using a series of guided images to portray the cancer cells being destroyed by healthy cells and by picturing the cancer shrinking. The visual process continues by imagining yourself well, free of disease and restored to health. Again, visualization is not an exercise in wishful thinking. Rather, it is a technique in changing your belief system about your illness and constantly reinforcing that belief system. Of course, visualization should be combined with the other self-help techniques (such as a healthy nutritional regime) to optimize its chances of working.

As Andrew Weil states in *Spontaneous Healing*, if you have doubts about the power of the mind to affect the body, pay attention to what happens to your body when you focus your mental or visual imagery in the realm of sexual fantasy! As Simonton has shown in *Getting Well Again* and, more recently, in his research center in the United States, one way in which visualization mobilizes the healing system is by healing damaged emotions. Visualization has the potential to help the auto immune system by reinforcing positive beliefs through mental images.

PAIN CONTROL

Many years ago I heard the old saying that pain is the body's warning signal that something somewhere is wrong. So it is clear that pain has a purpose. Of course, it is also true that psychological pain can be worse, far worse, than physical pain. Deep hurts cannot be as readily treated as physical pain. Further, they might worsen any physical pain you might be experiencing.

Psychological pain needs to be addressed if healing is to take place. Damaged emotions can, as already stated, act as a strong block to healing. You may need to talk to someone, either a close and trusted friend, or perhaps a health professional, such as a counselor, if you are hurting inside. Some people have told me that their cancers were opportunities to explore those painful things in their lives that they had suppressed for years. In this way, their cancers were opportunities for inner healing.

As far as physical pain is concerned, there are a few basic hints. The first is to report any pain to your doctor. Take any medication that she might prescribe but use it strictly as your doctor ordered. Make sure that your doctor closely monitors your pain, in order that the most effective treatment is given.

There are effective protocols for pain and you need not have to put up with a diminished quality of life. The breathing exercises outlined earlier in this chapter are also useful aids in minimizing pain. They help you to breathe through the pain, actually to 'break it down' into a 'momentary' sensation till it becomes manageable. Meditation is also a useful aid in pain control for both emotional and physical pain. This is so because pain is often linked to tension and fear. When you become deeply relaxed, your muscles loosen and the pain tends to diminish significantly. Note the visualization technique at the end of this book. Using a form of taped guided meditation can be particularly helpful. Talk about your pain. Those who communicate their pain with others find that this also helps.

KEEPING A JOURNAL

For very many years I have found writing a particularly therapeutic experience. If nothing else, it helps to externalize our feelings. Writing, in whatever form it takes, helps us to express our full range of emotions: our fears, our joys, our moods, our hopes and our doubts. A journey with cancer has many twists and turns, each having its own emotional response. A major illness such as this affects virtually every aspect of our life: our relationships, our work, our sexuality and our spirituality. It is therefore potentially a healing experience to make a record of this journey. The form this takes is entirely up to you. Keeping a diary allows you to view your problems in a more detached way.

I know some people who have expressed their emotions in the form of poetry. This is a healing experience because it lets you express your feelings, rather than suppress them. (Remember what we discussed in Chapter 3 about your emotions being translated into positive or negative chemical responses in your body.)

KEEPING YOUR LIFE IN BALANCE

This is another aspect of living with cancer that has been discussed extensively earlier in this book, especially in Chapters 2 and 3. It is important that you adhere to this principle and that you do not overdo things and thereby exhaust your body and depress your immune system. Since my diagnosis I have heard of a number of people who have taken a dramatic turn for the worse by not taking their illness into consideration. I recall a relatively young man who had liver cancer who insisted on continuing to work full-time in his business. He truly believed that he could manage a life-threatening illness and continue to run his business. Unfortunately, within a matter of three months his condition had deteriorated to the point where he was simply too ill to continue working.

I have also encountered a number of people who have gone on quite arduous overseas trips, which have also had a detrimental effect on the course of their illness. Long flights are very taxing on the immune system. Recycled air, the less than nutritious food served on aircraft and the effects of jet lag are not recommended. Keeping to a routine that includes things such as meditation, nutritious diet, juicing and supplementation are the staple ingredients of living well with cancer.

LAUGHTER AND MUSIC

Research has shown that laughter has psychological and physiological benefits. Laughter helps us deal with a range of emotions such as fear, anxiety and stress. At one group I attended the leader talked about the idea of 'laughing away your cancer.' It was certainly an interesting idea, however realistic or otherwise it may have been. At any rate, laughter has a positive effect on heart rate and blood pressure, it reduces pain and helps us to maintain a positive outlook.

In a similar way, music is something to which our systems seem to have been programmed. The potential of music to assist in healing body, mind and spirit is great. Music energizes our souls and stirs our emotions. It can calm us when we are annoyed or anxious, thus reducing our level of stress. Music can also inspire us with hope when we are sad or lonely. It can help to clear our minds and can act as a catalyst for releasing our creative energies. Pleasurable sounds tend to lift our spirits by taking us out of our situations and helping us to visualize a peaceful, happier environment. This is, of course, the logic of meditating to soft, pleasant music. (However music is not always an appropriate accompaniment to meditating as it can at times be distracting.)

Music and laughter provide us with positive, soothing thoughts and lift our mood. Our endorphins – the body's 'healing chemicals' – are increased in proportion to our psychological state. As these hormones are released into our bloodstreams, so our adrenalin levels drop. Stress and its by-product, muscular tension, are reduced. In turn, our immune functions are enhanced. Laughter and music also reduce our levels of cortisol, a steroid hormone associated with the adrenal complex. Stress raises the level of cortisol and, if prolonged, tends to exhaust our adrenal glands, thus lowering our immune responses. These are the main ways that music and laughter are therapeutic. Don't ignore their benefits.

SPIRITUALITY

This word is not necessarily related to commitment to a particular religion or set of religious doctrines. Spirituality means the ability to find peace in an imperfect world, and to feel that one's own personality is imperfect but acceptable. It also strongly suggests a reconnecting of the mind and the heart. I recognize, of course, that my definition is simplified and rather inadequate. Yet, in this context, it serves my purpose. Spirituality is reflected in a peaceful state of mind. What, then, are some of the ingredients of spirituality? Some of these were discussed in Chapter 2: acceptance, faith, forgiveness, peace and love are the main ingredients and seem to be present in long-term survivors. I would be a hypocrite if I were to suggest that it is easy to be 'spiritual' in the face of bad news, or when things are deteriorating. It is precisely at such times when we most need to 'let go' and 'let in' our understanding that suffering is not some random act of fate. It has an ultimate purpose that is unfortunately, at times, hidden from the limited view of our human perspective.

The proponents of biofeedback techniques, in which we learn to modify certain functions that are commonly thought of as involuntary, such as heart rate, skin temperature and a range of physiological functions, argue with a good deal of evidence that mind, body and emotions are a unitary system. This intriguing topic, discussed in Chapter 3, is mentioned again because of the huge importance that our mindsets, reflected in our lifestyles, can play in the course of our illnesses. A life-threatening illness demands that we give urgent attention to life's priorities. We need to do whatever it takes in our quest for wellness. Sometimes whatever it takes includes not only medical (whether conventional or unconventional) treatment, but also sorting through life's unfinished business. Issues such as getting rid of guilt, casting aside resentment and regret and righting those things which weigh on our consciences are an important part of achieving balance in our lives.

CHAPTER SUMMARY

- Problems relating to living with cancer fall into two categories: those related to treatment and those related to lifestyle.

- Unresolved emotional problems can be a causative factor in the onset of cancer.

- The trauma of a cancer diagnosis can exacerbate unresolved emotional problems. On the other hand, cancer can provide the opportunity to address the need for inner healing. Cancer can become a turning point – a re-evaluating of life's values and priorities. Your attitude to life is a vital determinant in the course of your illness.

- One of the chief causes of stress is fear. Fear has many causes. Take heart – note how each cause has a solution.

- Simple relaxation exercises provide a useful antidote to fear, anxiety and depression.

- Meditation – the silent healer can be used to help you recover. Meditation, along with visualization and creative imagery techniques can enhance your body's self-healing capacity.

- Pain is a problem that can always be alleviated. Follow your doctor's advice as well as the self-help techniques provided to help control pain.

- Writing as a means of self-expression is highly therapeutic.

- It is vital to keep your life in balance to help you on the road to recovery. Avoid excessive stress, such as long overseas journeys where possible. They have an adverse effect on your immune system.

- Laughter and music have strong healing properties. Make use of both of them.

- We are spiritual 'beings,' not human 'doings,' so take time to just 'be.'

ಓ 7 ಐ

HEALING YOUR LIFESTYLE

SOME YEARS AGO, WELL BEFORE I WAS DIAGNOSED WITH CANCER, I FOUND A BEAUTIFUL PRAYER ON THE BACK OF A CHURCH BULLETIN. This is a small extract from it:

> *We believe that we are immersed in mystery that our lives are more than they seem that we belong to each other and to a universe of great creative energies whose source and destiny is God...*

Suffering is of course not the only mystery of our lives. Cancer, like other major life events, forces us to reassess our lives. However, there is nothing like a life-threatening illness to bring us face to face with the meaning of life, to stop living according to other peoples' expectations and to start being the persons we really are. We need to embark on our healing journey not in a 'doing' mode but in a 'being' mode. In other words, in order to reach our full healing potential we need to give our wholehearted attention to getting well again not just because others may need us (however true this may be) but because we want to live the remainder of our lives purposefully, lovingly and authentically. Our faith and love can continue to grow no matter how damaged our bodies might become. Illness is far more than an unfortunate 'going wrong' of our bodies. Illness can be one of life's most powerful teachers. We need to learn to be still and to listen to its message. But how do we interpret the message of illness?

In another of his best-selling books, *Prescriptions for Living*, Dr. Bernie Siegel warns that guilt, blame and shame are never the appropriate responses to illness. Rather, you need to do everything possible in your quest to regain your health. The 'everything' includes learning about conventional and non-conventional treatments, as well as listening to the inner voice of your body. This is what Siegel calls the 'internal environment,' which he regards as a subtle yet awesome field of energy from which we still have much to learn. Siegel states that often this inner voice speaks as a symptom that mirrors our actions. I have found, as I am sure that many of my fellow cancer patients have also found, that my inner voice informs me where my illness fits into the larger pattern of my life.

I don't believe in coincidences. I believe that everything has a plan and a purpose – even a life-threatening illness. Occasionally we need to learn to be still, to learn the lessons of quietness and solitude to discover what that plan and purpose might be. Not infrequently that plan and purpose is not far beneath the surface of our lives. The short answer to my question of how to interpret the message of illness is to turn all of life's negativities into positives, challenges and opportunities.

Another way in which, paradoxically, cancer can help to heal your life is by choosing the way of wellness. By 'wellness' I refer to a harmony between body, mind and spirit. What you believe, the way you feel towards others, the things you say and do, all have an impact on your wellness. This holistic notion of wellness is something that can be independent of your physical condition. Your mental, emotional and spiritual health has a powerful effect on your well-being. Many cancer survivors have said that they considered their cancer to a 'wake-up call' to turn their lives around and mend those things which needed to be changed. It is in this respect that many cancer survivors have acknowledged the positive side to their illness. In many cases such people have, for the first time, taken personal responsibility for their lives. One of the common threads in the stories cancer patients recount about their healing journey is that their illness has not destroyed their wellness, but accomplished it. In some ways this is quite a remarkable thought, but absolutely true.

HOW TO ACHIEVE WELLNESS

- MAKE A DECISION TO LIVE WELL, EACH DAY REGARDLESS OF YOUR DIAGNOSIS, PROGNOSIS OR THE TREATMENT YOU ARE HAVING. You are not aiming merely to eliminate your physical symptoms. That is hardly a measure of wellness. Your aim is geared towards your total well-being, especially by nurturing your emotional and spiritual needs.

- MAKE WELLNESS YOUR AIM, REGARDLESS OF WHAT THE LENGTH OF YOUR LIFE MAY BE. You can do this only by focusing on the present; on living well each day, being thankful for the positive things that happen to you on a daily basis.

- TAKE PERSONAL RESPONSIBILITY FOR YOUR WELLBEING. Do not believe that your treatment alone can achieve your wellness. You must contribute to it. Regard the medical professionals who are treating you as your partners in healing, rather than as people who can bring about some kind of miracle cure.

- THE MEDICAL PROFESSIONALS WHO ARE TREATING YOU CAN BE CONCERNED WITH ONLY ONE PART OF YOUR HEALING – PRIMARILY THE MECHANICAL FUNCTIONS OF YOUR SYSTEM. It is up to you (perhaps with the assistance of a counselor) to mend your lifestyle in order to complete the healing process. Remember the lessons from Chapter 2, that the mind and the body form one unit. They are not separate. Your thoughts are chemical and affect the functioning of your body.

- ALWAYS LOOK ON THE BRIGHT SIDE OF LIFE – YOU WILL LIVE LONGER. (A recent long-term 30-year study conducted by the Mayo Clinic in Minnesota has concluded that pessimists have a 19 percent higher likelihood of premature death than optimists.)

- DEVELOP THE ATTITUDE THAT NOTHING IS MORE IMPORTANT IN YOUR LIFE THAN YOUR WORK OF ACHIEVING WELLNESS. Consider your priorities, then write down a daily schedule, which includes 'healing times' – times for meditation, prayer and listening to music. If you are still working, this task is even more important lest you crowd the day out and exclude time for yourself.

- MAKE SURE THAT YOUR WELLNESS ROUTINE INCORPORATES THE VARIOUS DIETARY RECOMMENDATIONS OUTLINED IN CHAPTER 4. A healthy diet, meditation and a positive attitude are the cornerstones of wellness. Don't fall into the trap of feeling that you have to change your diet. Choose to want to do this as part of your healing journey.

- INCLUDE EXERCISE AS PART OF YOUR 'WELLNESS' PROGRAM. Exercise is an important component of your new regime. Not only will it help you stay positive but also it will help with your energy levels as well. The type of exercise you do is your choice. Some people like to walk, others to swim or cycle, still others find a gentle exercise (which is really a moving meditation) such as tai chi to their liking.

- DON'T NEGLECT THE MATTER OF SUFFICIENT SLEEP. Some cancer therapies, particularly radiation and chemotherapy are debilitating. Therefore, it is a vital part of your healing that you have sufficient rest and sleep.

- FIND A POSITIVE SUPPORT GROUP. Don't go it alone. Support groups have two main functions: to provide social support and to provide information, especially on such matters as treatments and their side-effects, nutrition and a host of other lifestyle matters.

- LEARN TO EXPRESS YOUR EMOTIONS. Psychological research tells us that suppressing your emotions tends to weaken the immune system. Burying anger, guilt, shame, hurt and resentment is unhealthy and does nothing in the way of healing. To be able to forgive is to be able to let go of the past, with all its burdens. To forgive is to find peace of mind. Forgiving includes not only others but also yourself. Joan Borysenko, in her book *The Power of the Mind to Heal* (refer to Bibliography) has a particularly useful chapter on forgiveness and compassion. This chapter includes a forgiveness meditation that you may find very therapeutic.

- FIND A CHURCH, SYNAGOGUE, MOSK, A SPECIAL PLACE IN NATURE OR SOME OTHER PLACE OF WORSHIP WHERE YOU CAN FIND SPIRITUAL SUSTENANCE AND SUPPORT. Remember that the term spontaneous healing is a misnomer. Dramatic healings always tell us something about those who have experienced them. Often, those people have given equal consideration to their spiritual and emotional well-being, as to their physical welfare. In *Prescriptions for Living*, Dr. Bernie Siegel has a delightfully witty and powerful chapter called 'How Did I Get Here and May I Go Now? Thinking about God before disaster strikes.' Towards the end of this chapter Siegel writes:

> *When it is too much for you, say a prayer, leave it to God, and don't judge what God decides to do... If you want some direction, look to God – He's a great role model and coach. With the strength obtained through prayer, you can do God's work.*

- ALWAYS REMEMBER THAT THERE ARE WORSE THINGS THAT CAN HAPPEN TO YOU THAN A CANCER DIAGNOSIS. One writer has commented that cancer has both good and bad side-effects. Yes, good side-effects. Not infrequently, cancer can serve as a 'wake-up call' to redirect your life. (It did that for me.) It can repair damaged relationships, it can be a means of living more meaningfully and lovingly, treasuring each day as a gift and coming to terms with issues which have repeatedly been pushed into the background. One man told me not long ago that he was glad he had a cancer diagnosis and had not dropped dead from a heart attack. At least this way he is able to take stock of his life and make some changes.

- THE FACT THAT CANCER BRINGS US FACE TO FACE WITH OUR MORTALITY SHOULD BE SEEN AS A POSITIVE THING. After all, we are all going to die one day. Having a life threatening illness is a potent reminder to live well and not to waste our lives with things that ultimately do not matter. It also teaches us never to take our health for granted (as most people seem to do). At times your fears (dark clouds) will overshadow, or blot out your hopes and your peace of mind (the sunshine from your life). Take heart, this is also perfectly natural and is something we all go through.

THE IMPORTANCE OF LIVING IN THE PRESENT

Throughout this book, especially with reference to meditation, I have emphasized the importance of not 'awfulizing' about your illness. Don't be unduly influenced by what others say. One counselor with whom I spoke referred to 'toxic family and friends' – those whose influence makes us feel negative or fearful. You can't afford to be closely influenced by such people. It is so easy (and entirely understandable) to 'awfulize,' especially after a poor blood test or CT scan. We wonder if the downward trend can be reversed and our minds are flooded with fear. It is precisely at these times we would do well to remember the quote: 'Pessimism is a luxury I simply can't afford.'

Meditation and prayer – letting go of the burden of the past and the fear of the future (however problematic the present may be) – is the answer to coping with difficult situations. Each time you meditate you live in the present moment. This is a powerful de-stressor and protector of your immune system.

It is terribly important not to reinforce negative thought patterns. As stated earlier in this book daily positive affirmations are a valuable way of reinforcing positive messages to your subconscious mind. Never hesitate to seek help. Rearrange your priorities so that your needs at this important time are met.

CHAPTER SUMMARY

- Every case of cancer is unique. The common thread is that cancer can be viewed as a wake-up call to heal your life, to bring about an inner transformation.

- A sense of hopelessness can lower your immune function. Your positive attitude is an important part in the healing process.

- Stress management is a key technique in turning your life around. There are many ways to alleviate stress, including deliberately creating 'healing moments' or times of stillness in the day.

- Learn to live 'mindfully' in the present moment and not to project your fears into the future or to hang onto negative attitudes from the past.

- Meditation is strongly therapeutic. Research is growing that tends to support this idea.

- Try to keep your life in balance. Give yourself the opportunity to heal. Pay attention to mind, body and spirit in your quest for healing. We are spiritual beings as well as human beings.

ഇ 8 ര

REASONS FOR HOPE!

MY DIAGNOSIS TOOK PLACE UNDER UNFORTUNATE CIRCUMSTANCES. I had gone into hospital for minor surgery. During the course of that procedure the surgeon had discovered that I had 'widespread metastatic spread' (in other words, cancerous tumors) throughout my abdominal lining. Soon after I awoke, the surgeon rather bluntly informed me of his discovery. He told me that on the basis of what he saw I did not have much ground for hope – the cancer had already spread. He didn't believe that I had very long to live – probably months.

EXPLODING THE MYTHS

The suddenness and the rather dramatic circumstances of my diagnosis led me to see the myths of cancer, especially the first myth that the disease is universally fatal. In the light of the surgeon's prognosis I genuinely thought that I had only a few months left and that there was no cure and therefore no hope. I was more fearful of the process of dying than death itself. I recalled the awful suffering my father had experienced from prostate cancer twenty years earlier. Furthermore, I blamed myself for this unfortunate news. For a number of years I knew that my life was unbalanced. I wanted to change but simply kept shrugging it off. Silly as this may sound, there was a degree of self-blame and guilt for my diagnosis.

It was not too long before I had heard about people who had not only survived well beyond their prognosis, but also in some cases, had completely recovered from their illness. Amid the fear and anxiety of those early weeks and months, I discovered that I had real grounds for hope. Maybe I wasn't at the end of the road as the surgeon had predicted. After all, I had no pain and didn't feel particularly ill. I spoke to survivors and I read a book about those who had outlived their illness and had experienced remarkable recoveries. If they could do it, why couldn't I?

I began a strict dietary regime, began to meditate and use visualizations, and began a daily intake of vegetable juices. I also made other lifestyle changes. All of these aimed at cleansing my body and strengthening my immune system. Broadly speaking, my new routine aimed at meeting this serious challenge to my health and wellbeing. I was going to do everything possible to give my 'healing system' a chance to defy the odds and get well again. By 'healing system' I refer to that complex interaction of the various body systems, especially in the mind–body–spirit axis that Norman Cousins had discussed in his book *Anatomy of an Illness*.

I became aware that each case of remarkable recovery is unique. As I spoke to people who had recovered from cancer and as I read about such cases, I began to wonder why their doctors hadn't followed up such remarkable cases to try to determine what factors were responsible for their recoveries. In fact, I recognized a distinct pattern in such patients – a pattern that involved personality traits, beliefs, attitudes, social support, even moods and emotions. How did the doctors know that some or all of these traits were not as equally responsible for their patients' recovery as the chemotherapy, radiotherapy or whatever other medical treatment their patients had undergone? Did they put such recoveries down to spontaneous remissions? I believed then, as I believe now, that such 'non-medical' factors ought to be investigated and not merely relegated to the category of spontaneous remission. Could it not be that in some cases the mind–body components of such remarkable healing were as potent as the treatment given? My curiosity has increased in the last three years because my own cancer has, in the oncologist's words, 'not behaved in the way that it normally does.' Fortunately it has not gone on the course that my doctors had predicted, in spite of independent pathology reports that gave the diagnosis.

I regret the dividing wall of hostility between conventional and complementary medicine, recognizing of course, that change is difficult in a profession whose entire framework of acceptance is based on evidence from double-blind and randomized clinical studies. Nevertheless, I wondered why such scientific studies seemed to ignore such variables as: varying states of mind, individual health practices, social milieus, belief systems, religious experiences and so on. Don't these factors impinge on the progress of an illness such as cancer? How do the doctors know that it's not these non-scientific factors, these psycho-spiritual factors, rather than the treatment they had given, that is responsible for a patient's recovery? I felt that the medical profession should investigate more fully those cases of cancer that somehow just 'go away.'

CASES OF REMARKABLE RECOVERY

One of the many benefits of a support group is that we meet people who are really doing well and are defying the odds. The stories such people tell are a source of encouragement and hope. People who outlive their prognoses and who defy the odds are not endowed with huge doses of luck. Rather, they have worked hard at getting well again and have shown that their emotions really are chemical by the way they have prevailed over their illness. However, it would be overly simplistic and unfair to suggest that an indomitable spirit alone could, or does account for a 'remarkable recovery.'

Dr. Bernie Siegel's book *Love, Medicine and Miracles* profiles the characteristics of what he terms 'exceptional patients'– those who have made unexpected recoveries. They have, what he calls, 'survivor personalities.' They are worth remembering. Siegel states that such people usually have a measure of self-confidence about them and have a high degree of self-reliance. A patient he quotes in his book said that '...pessimism is a luxury I can't afford.' Resilience, adaptability and confidence are strong traits of survivor personalities. They are people who have come to terms with their lives, have found large measures of self acceptance and have measures of creativity. By creativity Siegel means looking at life creatively and seeing a cancer diagnosis as not the end but the beginning of a challenge – a challenge that certainly involves a reappraisal of life's goals and priorities.

Bernie Siegel, in his companion volume, *Peace, Love & Healing* also tells the story of a 78-year-old landscape gardener whom he had treated for stomach cancer, which normally has a poor prognosis. This man, John, had an amazingly positive outlook – full of optimism and sunshine, in spite of his serious illness. He delayed having surgery because it was spring – his busiest time of year. 'I want to make the world beautiful. That way if I survive, it's a gift. If I don't, I will have left a beautiful world,' he told Dr. Siegel during a consultation. A few weeks later John underwent surgery, healed remarkably rapidly and, despite a series of minor complications, his cancer eventually disappeared. Commenting on John's remarkable recovery, Dr. Siegel said, 'What you have to understand is that there is a biology of the individual as well as a biology of the disease, each affecting the other. On the day of diagnosis we don't know well enough to use a pathology report to predict the future.'

Perhaps the problem with those who recover when they are not expected to is that their recoveries are scientifically disreputable. They are regarded as statistical aberrations. What the medical profession needs to acknowledge is that the body's powerful self-healing capabilities can turn any illness (cancer included) around if it is given the right conditions. This is not for one moment to deny the vital importance of modern medicine. However, in cases such as my own, where conventional treatment had little to offer, I have managed to completely stabilize my illness by adopting a radically altered lifestyle that includes a wide range of natural remedies. As a doctor said to me not long ago in response to my wellness, 'It would seem you have made the soil of your body very inhospitable for your cancer to survive.'

Medical mysteries such as so-called spontaneous remissions are thought to happen by chance, yet the fact remains that there is much about the incredibly complex healing system that is not understood. The phrase 'spontaneous remission' is itself almost self-contradictory. Does the word remission mean something temporary or something permanent? Does spontaneous mean instantaneous? This phrase implies remission without a cause. Yet how could a disease such as cancer simply disappear? There must have been a reason for its disappearance.

In the early 1980's, Dr. Jeffrey Levin, an American immunologist, undertook a study of religion or spirituality and health outcomes. It was one of the first attempts to correlate religious belief and wellness scientifically. His findings, based on 250 case studies across various religious and ethnic groups, concluded that there was a 'protective effect of religious involvement.' This healing effect applied to a variety of diseases and included a range of religious affiliations. Levin's double blind clinical studies confirmed his findings. Cases of spontaneous remissions through prayer and deep faith (both on the part of those who are ill and those who care for them) have been reported throughout the world. I believe that faith is a powerful impetus to healing.

Ian Gawler, the co-founder of the Gawler Foundation in Victoria, Australia, was a young veterinary surgeon. In January 1975 he was diagnosed with a rare and usually fatal form of bone cancer, osteogenic sarcoma. His right leg was amputated. In November of the same year he had a recurrence and his condition deteriorated to the point that by March the following year he was thought to have only a matter of weeks to live. He had widespread secondaries (tumors) including bony lumps protruding on his chest. Gawler had an intensely strong will to live. He and his wife, Gayle, set about doing everything possible to help him recover. Gawler underwent conventional treatment (radiation therapy), as well as a range of unconventional therapies, including the Gerson diet, Filipino faith healers, massage, meditation and mental imagery. He devoted every waking hour to recovering. Gradually the tide turned. Dr. Ainslie Meares, the Melbourne psychiatrist who taught Gawler the healing art of meditation documented this extraordinary case of recovery in the *Medical Journal of Australia* (1978,2:433). Included in that report was the following:

The other important factor would seem to be the patient's state of mind. He has developed a degree of calm about him that I have rarely observed in anyone, even in oriental mystics ... When asked to what he attributes the regression of metastases he answers in some such terms as: 'I really think it is our way of life, the way we experience our life.' His extraordinarily low level of anxiety is obvious to the most casual observer. It is suggested that this has enhanced the activity of his immune system by reducing his level of cortisone.

In June 1978, Gawler was declared free of cancer. He has since helped thousands of people who have been touched by that illness. Many of those have achieved remarkable recoveries. Others have been helped to outlive their prognosis, while others again have been helped to improve the quality of their remaining time.

Some years ago a book was published called *Remarkable Recovery: What Extraordinary Healings Can Teach Us About Getting Well and Staying Well*. It was a book that explored the notion of 'remarkable recovery' from a wide variety of perspectives including the mind–body connection, the social connection and whether or not there might be such a thing as a 'recovery-prone' personality. This book, written by Carlyle Hirshberg, a biochemist, and Marc Barasch, a journalist was the product of a biochemist's database of 4,000 patients who had recovered from terminal illness. The chapter called 'The Miracle of Survival' probes the idea of the 'medical miracle' known commonly as spontaneous remission. The chapter begins with the description of an incident that took place at a cancer retreat.

It is a beautifully written and most inspiring piece of writing which shows us so much about the nature of healing. It also points to the fact that everyone needs to find and follow their own healing path.

The woman at the cancer retreat raised her hand. Pen poised over her small notebook, she announced, 'Okay, I'm ready – tell me everything I need to do to survive!'

The hope that glimmered in her dark eyes belied the anxious pull at the corners of her mouth. Caryle, who had just completed a talk on spontaneous remission, felt a slight flush of discomfort. She gave a sidelong, help-me glance to the medical director sitting to her right on the dais, but the doctor only smiled a faint smile that seemed to say, 'Well, well, let's see how you handle this one.'

Caryle had noticed the woman during the talk, furiously writing, looking up occasionally to assure herself she hadn't missed some critically important nuance. Looking out over the small group, she wondered, echoing the woman's query, 'What makes one person survive and another die? Are survivors the happy, enthusiastic types of current mind–body fable, or just the beneficiaries of a lucky role of the dice? How can anyone know until they are told, 'You have cancer' whether they will respond with despair or challenge, denial or attack?'

She slowly turned back to the woman and in a rose petal soft voice said the first thing that came to her mind. 'What you do must come from what you believe. I could give you every study, every list of everything associated with survival, but...,' and here she hesitated, groping for the right mixture of kindness and caution, 'these are still other people's solutions.'

Pausing to observe the effects of her words, discomfited by her own parsimony of prescription but knowing she was saying what was most true, she continued, 'I will give you that list, and you may find your answer. Or you may find it's like wearing someone else's well-worn shoes – they only sort of fit.'

The woman nodded, though her face betrayed a fleeting disappointment. But standard advice, no matter how careful or kindly, is of dubious value. Thinking of that roomful of people

128

who were either doing well, wished to, or might not, we began to wonder again about patterns: what is it that enables a person to survive great trauma, whether cancer or a life-shattering event? Crises come in many forms, whether critical illness, severe injury, war, imprisonment or abuse. The situations that overwhelm us arise from within our own bodies, from environment outside or, perhaps inevitably, from both.

One day we are whole. The next moment, all control is torn from our grasp. We may be flooded with fear of mortality, anger, or the strange crystalline calm of severe shock. But after shock ebbs comes a frightening burden of choice, made of equal parts instinct, experience and knowledge. A terminal diagnosis may be the end of the world to one person, a time to surrender to God for another, a call to battle for yet another. Crisis arouses the resources of the healing system, like a clamoring bell that awakens the sleeper; but such resources are channeled into different coping styles, whether inborn or learned. The goal, no matter what, is to gain mastery in a situation where lack of it could mean loss of life or sanity. The primeval urge to survive at almost any cost is at the root of the organism's response to challenge.

From this short chapter, I hope it has become clear that recovery from cancer or any other life-threatening illness has an element of mystery attached to it, while at the same time having much rational explanation. The very notion of spontaneous remission is mysterious. Over and again, the question is asked, 'Why do some experience this, while others do not?' It seems possible that the reason spontaneous remissions occur is that the body's natural defense system is stimulated to help overcome the cancer. Because spontaneous remissions are not documented in the medical literature, we rely on hearsay and anecdotal reports. The fact remains that such remissions from illness do occur, and probably more frequently than is commonly acknowledged.

There is an important difference between spontaneous remission and long-term survival. The former is quite unpredictable while the latter is generally associated with radical lifestyle changes.

CHAPTER SUMMARY

- Do not allow the shock of the diagnosis allow you to 'awfulize.' Imprint as many positive and hopeful affirmations into your subconscious as possible.

- People have recovered from cancer; it is not an uncommon occurrence.

- Every case of 'remarkable recovery' or spontaneous remission has its unique set of circumstances.

- No one knows whether the mind–body component of a cancer recovery is as strong as the actual (conventional) treatment or not.

- Cases of remarkable recovery are a valuable source of inspiration and hope.

- Dr. Bernie Siegel's 'survivor personalities,' as described in *Love, Medicine and Miracles* are important, inspirational role models.

- There is much about the complex 'healing system' that is simply not understood.

- There are important differences between spontaneous remission and long-term survivors.

&

ADDITIONAL MATERIALS

℘ Appendix One ℃

FREQUENTLY ASKED QUESTIONS

A CANCER DIAGNOSIS BRINGS WITH IT INNUMERABLE QUESTIONS. These include the course of the illness, life expectancy, treatment options, side effects, lifestyle questions, and so on. The common denominator of these questions is survival. We want to know how best to optimize our chances. We want to have some degree of control over our situation. We want to maintain our quality of life. We want to give our lives meaning. The following questions and answers attempt to cover a few of the more common concerns that people have after a cancer diagnosis.

What is the most important overall advice you could give to someone who has just learned that they have cancer?

The first thing you should do is to seek out the best possible medical practitioner who has had extensive experience successfully treating your type of cancer. This may involve getting a second opinion, especially if the suggested treatment is radical. After you have decided on a course of treatment, be an active participant in it. Believe that it will help you to get well again. Adapt your lifestyle to give your treatment the best possible chance of success. Remember that you need to 'do whatever it takes' to overcome a life-threatening illness. You cannot expect to turn your illness around with a passive approach. You must participate in your own cure and be willing to meet the challenge of beating this disease. Use the best that conventional and complementary treatments have to offer.

How useful is the Internet as a source of information?

The Internet is an excellent resource for contacting people for information and support. By all means make full use of it but you need to evaluate carefully the source of whatever information you find. Use your judgment as to the reliability of the source. The Internet can be a very useful way of being put in touch with others who have your type of cancer. You can find out their experiences with different types of treatments.

To what extent can a person's mental and emotional make-up affect the outcome of their disease?

As suggested throughout this book, your emotions are chemical. Your attitudes and beliefs have physiological effects. In many traditional cultures, when a curse or death charm was placed on someone, he often became ill and died within a fairly short period of time. The same can be true after a cancer diagnosis. If a doctor tells a patient that she only has a short time to live, that knowledge can easily become imprinted on the subconscious mind, become a part of that person's belief and, indeed, hasten that person's death. Having a positive attitude is a choice – a simple but profound choice. Once that choice is made, you need to act upon it and do everything in your power to make sure that you end up on the 'right side of the statistics.' Being hopeful about the outcome of your illness is actually part of being positive. Whatever the outcome of your illness might be, the most important thing is to live in the present and have a meaningful existence. Remember that all of us are in 'terminal' conditions. The important thing is how we use the time we have left. There is a sense in which having a cancer diagnosis is a positive experience because it confronts us with mortality and forces us to reassess life's priorities.

How does a person get their life back together after the initial shock of the diagnosis?

This is a difficult question to answer because everyone's situation is different. Certainly in a hospital situation you have little control. Once you are beyond that stage and have commenced a course of treatment you will have more control over your life. One of the things that help you get that control is to acquire as much information as you possibly can and be part of the decision making process. Adopting some of the self-help techniques, especially meditation and visualization, goes a long way to helping you regain control of your life. Participate in your endeavor to regain your wellness. The power of the mind is very powerful. This is scientifically proven and positive thinking changes the biochemistry of the body. Your treatments should be meditated upon as both in positive imagery and in contemplation. Whatever problems and questions worry you, talk and ask about them at every opportunity. Participate in your endeavor to regain your wellness. Don't be merely a passive recipient of treatment.

How does a person decide whether or not to use complementary or unconventional therapies?

Do not be unduly influenced by any publication that has the term 'cancer cure' on its cover. There are numerous so-called cures for cancer. Unfortunately, these cures seem to rest their cases more on anecdotal responses than on any scientific evidence. While it is important to speak to patients who have undergone the therapy you are considering, do not be too strongly influenced by anecdotal evidence. Likewise, beware of well-intentioned friends or family members who come up with cancer cures. If you are interested in a non-conventional treatment regime, first find out what evidence is available regarding its rate of success. Find out about its cost and duration and, most importantly, whether it has been successfully used for your type of cancer. Find out whether there is any risk of toxicity or harm from the therapy in question.

Finally, ask your doctor whether the proposed treatment might interact with any other treatment you are having. There are a number of complementary therapies, especially herbal, mineral and vitamin supplements I believe can greatly assist most cases of cancer and their treatments, especially chemotherapy and radiotherapy. Speak to a holistic medical practitioner or a qualified medical herbalist about this.

How would you describe the relationship between hope and survival?

The connection between hope and survival serves to illustrate the interconnectedness between medicine, psychology and spirituality. The unfortunate thing is that the majority of doctors have time to be concerned only about the patient's illness. So many are unaware that the level of illness can be, to a considerable degree, a barometer of the person's state of mind. Our medical system is not geared to take a holistic view of disease.

In his book *Peace, Love and Healing* Dr. Bernie Siegel states that anything that offers hope has the potential to heal, including thoughts, suggestions, symbols and placebos. These things cannot, therefore, be thought of as giving false hope because hope is entirely a subjective experience. It is not based on any one external criterion. Faith and trust give substance to hope. It is only when we take responsibility for our lives that we learn to trust. We need to trust that healing is taking place, although at times this healing may be inner healing and not necessarily the healing of the body. Hope, without any affirmation of it in our day-to-day living, is not hope but rather wishful thinking. Hope must be expressed in our thoughts and in every aspect of our lives. This is the meaning of saying that people heal from within. Faith, hope, love, laughter and acceptance are integral qualities of surviving an illness such as cancer.

In what ways does love actually help in the healing process?

Dr. Candace Pert's book *Molecules of Emotion* explains in scientific terms how neuro-transmitters send neuro-peptides from the base of the pituitary gland throughout our bloodstreams in accordance with our states of mind. She has scientifically investigated the connection between our minds and the functioning of our bodies. She and others have shown that love, especially unconditional love, has the capacity to enhance the healing process. Love and healing are always possible, irrespective of whether or not a cure eventuates. Unconditional love, especially for one who has been touched by cancer, is very important. Many people are strangers to unconditional love – love with no strings attached. This is why their emotional growth is stunted. Guilt, fear, anxiety and depression, the great enemies of love, have at times contributed to a person's cancer. A negative mindset adversely affects the body's healing system. That is why it is important to allow yourself to love (and that includes self-love) and be loved.

Is love something that all of us can attain, even if we live solitary lives?

Love is an innate gift to humankind. Sadly this gift is not given to some individuals in their childhood or beyond and their life is blighted and disfigured as a result.

People define God in different ways. Some refer to God as a creative intelligence, as in our body's innate ability for self-healing. A prime example of this is when we cut our fingers or graze our knees. We don't need to do anything beyond washing the wounds. We heal naturally. Others believe in a personal God who revealed Himself in the Bible and who lives by faith in the hearts of those who believe and trust Him. Others still, experience God in the beauty of nature. In other words, love takes many different forms. However we interpret God and love we need to take account of self-acceptance and self-love. This is a most important precondition of healing. Your cancer is not a punishment for anything in life that you may have done. God is an ever-present resource – whatever our circumstances. That is why we need to accept ourselves as we are. Then we can come to be right with our God. Thornton Wilder once said that there is a land of the living and a land of the dead, and if the bridge is love, then we will all survive. This means that if you want to be immortal, love somebody; then a part of you lives forever. True, isn't it? If loneliness, isolation and a sense of alienation is burdening you, seek out someone with whom you can relate. Join a support group. This is certainly one place where unconditional love and acceptance is freely available. In doing this you will certainly enhance your healing capacity.

Is it possible to recover from all types of cancer?

The answer to this is a resounding 'yes,' even if your cancer has spread and you have developed secondary tumors. Read accounts of people who have survived and are leading normal lives if you need to be convinced about this matter. A growing number of people with cancer have beaten the odds and recovered from very difficult medical situations. Ironically, many of these survivors report that cancer has ultimately improved their quality of life.

What are the key characteristics of long-term survivors?

In summary, they are the people who fill their lives with 'live' messages. They are people who live life to the full and have learned to live in the present moment and make a commitment to living. Long-term survivors tend to be those people who have learned to achieve balance and order in their lives. They are people who have learned to shake off regrets, resentments and negativity and replace them with faith, hope, love and laughter.

Another characteristic of long-term survivors is that they don't go it alone, they get support and find people to share with:

family, friends and a support group. Cancer survivors have taken an active role in their own wellness. They have sought out the best advice and the most appropriate treatment regime. Often they also use some form of complementary treatment, such as vitamin, mineral or herbal supplements, or perhaps they juice regularly. They are aware of the spiritual dimension of their lives and nurture their spirituality. They have faced up to mortality and are not afraid of death.

✂ Appendix Two ✂

YOUR RIGHTS AS A PATIENT

In the aftermath of a cancer diagnosis, with all of its accompanying trauma, it is easy to lose sight of the fact that not only do you have choices, but also you have a legal right to sign or not to sign a consent form to treatment. Some patients believe that they have no right to question a doctor's advice. Sometimes the problem is that in their sense of desperation they forget that there are important matters over which they have some choice.

On an apparently less 'practical' level is the matter of how you perceive your illness. Near the beginning of her book *Quest for Life*, Petrea King highlights this issue. After relating her own feelings of powerlessness and depression following her leukaemia diagnosis, she explained that a simple change of perception made a vast difference to the way she experienced this adversity. She wrote:

One set of thoughts brought depression and a distinct feeling of powerlessness, whilst another brought a sense of hope and positiveness. We can't always change the outcome of a disease but we can change the way in which we can experience that outcome.

The most important factor that determines your decision regarding treatment options is your understanding of what is involved and your knowledge of the particular treatment's chance of success and side-effects. It might be a good idea to have another look at the checklist of questions you should ask your doctor. Self-empowerment, not powerlessness, is an important pre-requisite to healing but you need to have enough information regarding the treatments being offered you. If your doctor offers you no hope, then find another doctor. Even in a difficult medical situation, when the prognosis looks bleak, hope should never be taken away.

While it is most important that you have a good rapport with your doctor and you place your trust in his expertise, you also need to remember that it is your life that is being discussed. To have an inner conviction that the treatment is right for you is most important. Your intuitive feelings should not be ignored. A negative perception of a treatment stands in the way of your body's ability to respond favorably.

CONSENTING TO TREATMENT

By law, most procedures these days need your consent. As the patient, you should be given a full understanding of what is involved in the proposed treatment. It is your right to refuse the recommended treatment. No one, however well informed, has the right to put you under duress. You should never surrender your control – with the exception of being an accident victim waiting for an ambulance. You have a right to refuse treatment, especially when your quality of life could be severely compromised. Sometimes there may be an alternative treatment available. It is your life and your decision. Family members and medical practitioners need to respect your integrity and independence. Only you can make the decision whether or not your life is worth living and in what circumstances. If you have any question about your legal rights as a patient you should consult with an attorney.

SUMMARY

- Do not be a 'passive patient.' You have the right of choice and only you can make a decision based on the best possible advice.

- The way you perceive your illness is a critical variable in your capacity to recover.

- Your doctor should explain the options to you. You may share the choice you make with her.

- Try to read as much as you can about a proposed treatment. Don't be rushed into making a decision, unless there is an obvious urgency about the matter.

℘ Appendix Three ℧

AUTHOR'S PRAYERS
FOR HOPE & FAITH

PSALM 23

The Lord is my shepherd, I shall not want;
He makes me lie down in green pastures,
He leads me beside still waters;
He restores my soul.
He leads me in paths of righteousness for his name's sake.
Even though I walk through the valley of the shadow of death
I fear no evil –for thou art with me,
Your rod and thy staff they comfort me.
You prepare a table before me in the presence of my enemies;
You anoint my head with oil, my cup overflows.
Surely goodness and mercy shall follow me
all the days of my life.
And I shall dwell in the house of the Lord for ever.

PEACE PRAYER

Lord, make me an instrument of your peace.
Where there is hatred, let me sow love.
Where there is injury, pardon.
Where there is doubt, faith.
Where there is despair, hope.
Where there is darkness, light,
Where there is sadness, joy.
Divine Master, grant that I may not so much seek
To be consoled, as to console;
To be understood, as to understand;
To be loved, as to love;
For it is in giving that we receive,
It is in pardoning that we are pardoned,
It is in dying that we are born to eternal life.

ST. FRANCIS OF ASSISI

℘ Appendix Four ℘

WORDS OF WISDOM FROM BERNIE SIEGEL, M.D.

Bernie Siegel, M.D. is one of the world's foremost physicians, authors, motivational speakers and advocates for individuals facing the challenges of chronic illnesses. He is the founder of Exceptional Cancer Patients (ECaP) and the author of Love, Medicine and Miracles, Peace, Love and Healing, How to Live Between Office Visits, and many other inspirational books and articles.

Several years ago, we were very fortunate to have Dr. Siegel speak to our patient community. Dr. Siegel's insights and teachings are not just inspirational but provide a fresh way to look at life with all its challenges. The entire teleconference was digitally recorded and is available for listening at our website.

Here are some excerpts and quotes from Dr. Siegel's discussion:

Doctors:

- An enormous part of the problem is so called medical education. It's not an education. It's information. You are not taught how to take care of people

- If you write the word "words words words" with no space between them you realize it becomes sword, sword, sword. The point is that we can kill people with our words and we are not trained how to communicate.

- We really need to change the process in medical schools.

- Good doctors will accept criticisms from patients, family, and nurses. Good doctors learn from those around them.

- Medicine needs to study success.

Survival:

- Beating cancer to me is about your attitude towards life and cancer and your mortality.

- Personality has a lot to do with long term survival. These are people who had meaning in their life, expressed anger appropriately, asked for help when they needed it, said no to things they don't want to do. They used their feelings to improve their life, rather than get depressed.

- Our body chemistry affects are genes. You can't separate yourself from your life experience because it becomes your chemistry.

- Information doesn't change anyone. You need inspiration to go with the information.

- Do what you love so that you serve the world in your way, not a way imposed by others.

- Death isn't a failure. We are all going to run out of time some day. The important thing is to live.

Patients:

- If anyone has to go to the hospital you should take what I call the "Siegel Kit" which is a magic marker, a noise maker, and a water gun. If you ever go to the operating room, you write "not this one stupid" and "cut here." So

146

they don't make mistakes and you can put a few other comments so that the surgeon smiles when he sees the notes you have written on your body. That way you become a human being. You want a noise maker so that when you really need help and you push the call button and nobody shows up, you make noise. And you want a water gun so that if anyone enters your room when you've shut the door, because you want some quiet time to meditate, play or sit with your family, you take out the water gun and squirt them. That empowers you. They won't forget you and it will help you get special treatment.

✃ Appendix Five ✃

CANCERWIRE INTERVIEW

Surviving Mesothelioma, a Terminal Cancer:
Paul Kraus' Remarkable Story
© Cancer Monthly 2005

This interview originally appeared in the
March 2005 edition of CancerWire

For anyone faced with a dire prognosis of cancer or any other disease, the following interview will inspire you. In the annals of cancer, mesothelioma is one of the worst possible types of cancer to have. In the words of oncologists it has a "dismal therapeutic outcome"[1] and is "an aggressive incurable tumor."[2] The median survival from diagnosis ranges from 6 to 18 months.[3] Despite this prognosis, Mr. Paul Kraus is alive many years after he was diagnosed with peritoneal mesothelioma. What is equally remarkable is that Mr. Kraus had no orthodox cancer therapies – he opted to say 'no' to chemotherapy, surgery, and radiation. Instead, Mr. Kraus made radical lifestyle changes, altering his diet, using intravenous and oral vitamins, herbs, amino acids and other immune boosting therapies and supplements, and tapping into the power of the mind-body connection.

---

[1] *Phase II trial of a single weekly intravenous dose of ranpirnase in patients with unresectable malignant mesothelioma.* Mikulski SM, et al., J Clin Oncol. 2002 Jan 1;20(1):274-81.
[2] *A multicentre phase II study of cisplatin and gemcitabine for malignant mesothelioma.* Nowak AK, et al., Br J Cancer. 2002 Aug 27;87(5):491-6.
[3] *A multicentre phase II study of cisplatin and gemcitabine for malignant mesothelioma.* Nowak AK, et al., Br J Cancer. 2002 Aug 27;87(5):491-6.

The Diagnosis

Cancer Monthly: Paul can you tell us when you were diagnosed and what types of symptoms you experienced that led to your diagnosis?

PK: I was diagnosed at the end of June 1997. The only symptom I had was a very bloated abdomen. I did not have any pain. I actually went into the hospital for an umbilical hernia repair and the cancer was an accidental finding. During the surgery the surgeon removed a lot of fluid from my abdomen. He also conducted a laparoscopic examination that revealed widespread metastases. He first thought that I had metastatic pancreatic cancer. It took two or three weeks for the pathology to come back from Sydney and say that in fact it was mesothelioma.

Cancer Monthly: And that diagnosis was reconfirmed by another hospital?

PK: Yes, my pathology was sent to Australia's leading pathologist in mesothelioma cases, Professor Douglas Henderson of Adelaide. They had two teams of pathologists verify and confirm the diagnosis. In fact, it was confirmed as peritoneal or abdominal rather than pleural mesothelioma. This is a very unusual subtype, even within the annals of mesothelioma.

Cancer Monthly: Does peritoneal mesothelioma have the same kind of dire prognosis as the more frequently encountered pleural mesothelioma?

PK: Yes. In fact, when we first went to a professor of oncology in Sydney, we thought that peritoneal is less dangerous than pleural. He shook his head and said, "Oh, no, oh no. In fact, in some ways it is even more difficult."

149

Cancer Monthly: How was your health history prior to that diagnosis?

PK: It had been good, but I had suffered from a lot of stress. And there were minor family traumas in the previous 12 to 18 months before diagnosis. Some writers say that things like that may affect one's immune function. Sometimes I conjecture whether that was a little warning or a tap on the shoulder from someone upstairs to change my lifestyle, which I of course I radically did, but more about that in a few minutes.

Previous Exposure to Asbestos

Cancer Monthly: Now, mesothelioma regardless of the subtype is associated with prior exposure to asbestos. Had you been exposed to asbestos?

PK: For the first 12 or 18 months after my diagnosis I did not make the connection that about 35 years earlier I had been exposed to asbestos. I am a former high school teacher. I did not work with asbestos in any way. But, in the early 1960's when I was a university student and on my vacation, I was working in a factory where they were sawing asbestos fiber sheets nearby. There, I was exposed to that blue dust for a few weeks. Nobody warned me. There were no warnings, no signs. This was the only known source of exposure for me. After leaving university I became a high school teacher and a writer. So I had no other known exposure. In fact, my early medical records stated that this patient has no known exposure to asbestos. The disease lay dormant for all that time.

Cancer Monthly: Did you file suit?

PK: I did eventually take up proceedings (sue). I was very very reluctant to do this. In fact I flatly refused. However, I was prompted by my son. He pointed out correctly what this diagnosis has done to my life. How my income had been slashed, and so on. I finally succumbed to these promptings and succeeded in gaining compensation for my damages.

Treatment Choices

Cancer Monthly: Now, you are faced with this horrible diagnosis and I imagine you are being offered perhaps surgery, chemotherapy or radiation. Instead you opted not to have any orthodox treatments. Can you tell us how you came to make these decisions?

PK: Actually, I was not offered much hope at all. My medical prognosis was very poor. At that time, I asked what were the chances of success with chemotherapy and I was told not very high at all. That's why I opted for a different path. Apart from being racked with fear and the fact that the fluid in my abdomen was building up again, I did not have any pain. My quality of life was, at that moment, okay. I made the decision not to go down that so called conventional path because I was told by the doctors that my quality of life would be quite severely compromised with the heavy chemotherapy I would have been prescribed. And so I made a major decision. I decided to radically change my lifestyle. I read books by Bernie Siegel (Peace, Love and Healing: Bodymind Communication & the Path to Self-Healing: An Exploration; Love, Medicine and Miracles: Lessons Learned about Self-Healing from a Surgeon's Experience with Exceptional Patients). I read books by Andrew Weil (Spontaneous Healing), and Simonton and Matthews (Getting Well Again). These books were incredibly inspirational and useful. For example, Andrew Weil wrote that any illness can be conquered through radical lifestyle change because our bodies are made with powerful self-healing capacities. It was damn hard to make such radical changes, but I was determined to see them through. I realized that to do otherwise meant that my chances of surviving were greatly diminished.

I made the decision that I am going to do everything I possibly can to turn this illness around. I began juicing --- carrot juice and beetroot juice, as well as green juices four or five times a day. I learned to meditate and use visualization. I did this for hours. I also prayed. I went to prayer groups and healing groups. I learned affirmations. I radically altered my diet into a vegetarian diet. I cut-out sugar. I ate high-fiber, predominantly raw food, but not exclusively. I also focused on exercise. I began taking vitamin, mineral, herbal and homeopathic supplements along with amino acids (N-Acetyl-Cystine (NAC), methylcobalamin, reduced glutathione). Also I took vitamins A, C, and E. Non-acidic vitamin C. Calcium ascorbate powder. I take slightly less now than I what I did initially. For the first couple of years after the diagnosis I was taking 8 grams a day in divided doses of Vitamin C in the form of calcium ascorbate.

Cancer Monthly: Were you taking the Vitamin C orally or intravenously.

PK: I took the 8 grams orally, it's in powder form and I dissolved it in water. But one of the therapies that I count as very important in those early days was the intravenous vitamin C that I had administered in conjunction with what is called ozone therapy.

Cancer Monthly: And how was the ozone therapy administered?

PK: Intravenously. They took blood out of a vein, used an ozone machine to ozone the blood and reintroduced it into my body through a drip. The rationale for that was that cancer does not like an oxygenated environment and the ozone therapy greatly helped to oxygenate the cells. In addition, I used another treatment when I was first diagnosed called Ukrain. These treatments were an adjunct to my lifestyle change.

The other thing I should say that I think is terribly important, almost fundamental, is that for the first four or five months after diagnosis, the volume of fluid in my abdomen was not really improving. I complained to my doctor, I said, "Look I'm doing all this and nothing is happening." And he reminded me, admonished me actually, and he said, "Be patient because this takes time. You are getting better. You affirm that you are getting better in your affirmations and your visualizations which you use in conjunction with these therapies. So just give it time." And he was right. His words were prophetic. They did in fact stabilize my cancer.

Cancer Monthly: For the treatments you mentioned, the Ukrain, ozone therapy, Vitamin C, supplements, other vitamins, how were you able to put that regimen or protocol together? Did you find it all in one place or in parts from your research and reading?

PK: This protocol or regime came about from my intensive research. I did not have access to the internet at that stage, back in 1997, but a friend did. We researched it together. Also, I had by great fortune a holistic doctor, a general practitioner. He routinely used intravenous C for other cancer patients. That particular aspect of the protocol was through him. He also said he had heard about Ukrain but that he did not know very much about it. So we tracked it down and incorporated it into my treatment and the same with the ozone therapy. He had said that he did not know too much about ozone therapy but that in my situation it was worth a try.

Cancer Monthly: That's absolutely fantastic that you had an open-minded holistic practitioner who was willing to try things with you.

PK: Yes.

Cancer Monthly: In terms of the timeline, did you start this protocol soon after your diagnosis or was there a period where you waited? How quickly did you start all of this?

PK: The radical lifestyle change especially regarding diet, I started virtually immediately. The juicing and changing of my diet to the vegetarian, low fat, no sugar I started literally within a few days of being diagnosed. Now for the supplements, within a month I was on the basic vitamins A, C, and E. Then gradually over the first few months after that I learned about some of these minerals such as selenium which is a very important and the amino acids and so on. I started on intravenous C within 6 weeks of diagnosis. And I learned to meditate. I was reading the books that I mentioned earlier within a couple of weeks after I was diagnosed.

Cancer Monthly: How are you doing now?

PK: I feel fine. I live day to day. My tests are okay. They say that I still have cancer and my energy level is not very good. But, I'm fine. I don't have any pain. My doctor tells me, "You're fine. Just keep up what you are doing and you will go on for years." He's convinced of it because the CT scans do not show any deterioration. They do vary a bit. They do show there is still fluid, but I have affirmed that sure there's fluid in there but it's probably non-malignant by now.

Cancer Monthly: And from the time of your diagnosis until now you have never had chemotherapy, radiation, or surgery?

PK: That is correct. In fact in August 2000, I was under a great deal of stress because one of my children was very ill. My condition began to deteriorate and I saw an eminent cancer surgeon. He recommended that I have a very major surgery. What is called a peritonectomy where they remove, over 10 or 12 hours, the entire peritoneal lining. And I really meditated on that, I thought about it. I asked my general practitioner about it.

154

He said, "Look even though the test shows a deterioration, how are you feeling?" I said, "I feel fine. I don't have any pain." He said, "Go back on the intravenous C. Go back on the Ukrain. Go back on the ozone therapy." And he felt confident that since I had done it once before I could do it again. And he was right. So I did not have surgery.

Cancer Monthly: So you went back on the protocol in August 2000 and stayed on it for how long?

PK: About 14 or 15 months. I know if this happens again I'll just return to that full IV protocol.

Cancer Monthly: And now you are doing what one might call maintenance therapy?

PK: That's exactly right.

Cancer Monthly: And that's comprised of the oral vitamins, minerals, other supplements, and diet?

PK: That is correct.

Mind & Body Connection

Cancer Monthly: You have talked about the importance of the regimen and also the importance of a positive mental state. Would you say that your mental state is as essential as the therapies?

PK: Absolutely. I would be giving a false impression if I were to say I was psychologically on top of things from the beginning. I was not, especially in the first six months after diagnosis. At that point, it was not so much a struggle against cancer as it was a struggle with myself, with my constant fears and doubts. That was my battle. I was battling myself as much as I was the cancer. There is something terribly important here.

As part of my therapy, I wrote a journal which ultimately became a book called Faith, Hope, Love and Laugher: How They Heal. It was highly therapeutic in my case just writing down thoughts and fears and doubts; chronicling these sorts of things.

Also, I'll never forget the first day that I had those intravenous therapies administered. I was very fearful. The nurse who was doing the administrating detected my fears. She put everything down and said, "I want you to affirm, visualize as I administer these therapies that they are actually doing you good. This is very important and powerful to your healing. If you don't accept that these therapies are doing you good then the treatment will not work because your mind and your body are one." She was right. The mind body connection is very important for healing. They are inextricably linked. If one has the wrong attitude one cannot be a survivor of mesothelioma or any form of cancer.

ဆ Appendix Six ଔ

MESOTHELIOMA PRIMER

Mesothelioma is a rare form of cancer in which malignant (cancerous) cells are found in the mesothelium, a protective sac that covers most of the body's internal organs.

What is the mesothelium?

The mesothelium is a membrane that covers and protects most of the internal organs of the body. It is composed of two layers of cells: One layer immediately surrounds the organ; the other forms a sac around it. The mesothelium produces a lubricating fluid that is released between these layers, allowing moving organs (such as the beating heart and the expanding and contracting lungs) to glide easily against adjacent structures.

The mesothelium has different names, depending on its location in the body. The peritoneum is the mesothelial tissue that covers most of the organs in the abdominal cavity. The pleura is the membrane that surrounds the lungs and lines the wall of the chest cavity. The pericardium covers and protects the heart.

What is mesothelioma?

Mesothelioma (cancer of the mesothelium) is a disease in which cells of the mesothelium become abnormal and divide without control or order. They can invade and damage nearby tissues and organs. Cancer cells can also metastasize (spread) from their original site to other parts of the body. Most cases of mesothelioma begin in the pleura or peritoneum.

157

How common is mesothelioma?

About 3,000 new cases of mesothelioma are diagnosed in the United States each year. Mesothelioma occurs more often in men than in women and risk increases with age, but this disease can appear in either men or women at any age.

What are the risk factors for mesothelioma?

Exposure to asbestos is the major risk factor for mesothelioma. A history of asbestos exposure at work is reported in the majority of cases.

What is asbestos?

Asbestos is the name of a group of minerals that occur naturally as masses of strong, flexible fibers that can be separated into thin threads and woven. Asbestos has been widely used in many industrial products, including cement, brake linings, roof shingles, flooring products, textiles, and insulation. If tiny asbestos particles float in the air, they may be inhaled or swallowed, and can cause serious health problems. In addition to mesothelioma, exposure to asbestos increases the risk of lung cancer, asbestosis (a non-cancerous, chronic lung ailment), and other cancers, such as those of the larynx and kidney.

Who is at increased risk for developing mesothelioma?

Because asbestos was used in so many products, millions of Americans have been exposed to asbestos dust. An increased risk of developing mesothelioma was originally found among shipyard workers, people who work in asbestos mines and mills, producers of asbestos products, workers in the heating and construction industries, and other trades people. Today, mesothelioma victims include many people exposed to asbestos at home or from the clothes of a loved one who worked with

158

asbestos containing products. The U.S. Occupational Safety and Health Administration (OSHA) sets limits for acceptable levels of asbestos exposure in the workplace. People who work with asbestos wear personal protective equipment to lower their risk of exposure.

If you have been diagnosed with mesothelioma there is a very high statistical chance that you have been exposed to asbestos at some time (or multiple times) in your life.

What are the symptoms of mesothelioma?

Symptoms of mesothelioma may not appear until 30 to 50 years after exposure to asbestos. Shortness of breath and pain in the chest due to an accumulation of fluid in the pleura are often symptoms of pleural mesothelioma. Symptoms of peritoneal mesothelioma may include weight loss and abdominal pain and swelling due to a buildup of fluid in the abdomen. If the cancer has spread beyond the mesothelium to other parts of the body, symptoms may include pain, trouble swallowing, or swelling of the neck or face.

How is mesothelioma diagnosed?

Diagnosing mesothelioma is often difficult, because the symptoms are similar to those of a number of other conditions. Diagnosis begins with a review of the patient's medical history. A complete physical examination may be performed, including x-rays of the chest or abdomen and lung function tests. A CT (or CAT) scan or an MRI may also be useful. A biopsy confirms a diagnosis of mesothelioma. In a biopsy, a surgeon or a medical oncologist removes a sample of tissue for examination under a microscope by a pathologist.

Mesothelioma is described as localized if the cancer is found only on the membrane surface where it originated. It is classified as advanced if it has spread beyond the original membrane surface to other parts of the body, such as the lymph nodes, lungs, chest wall, or abdominal organs.

159

What is the conventional approach to treating mesothelioma?

Treatment for mesothelioma depends on the location of the cancer, the stage of the disease, and the patient's age and general health. Standard treatment options include surgery, radiation therapy, and chemotherapy. Sometimes, these treatments are combined. Standard treatment for all but localized mesothelioma is generally not curative.[1]

Surgery - Extrapleural Pneumonectomy in selected patients with early stage disease may improve recurrence-free survival, but its impact on overall survival is unknown. Pleurectomy and decortication can provide palliative relief from symptomatic effusions, discomfort caused by tumor burden, and pain caused by invasive tumor. Operative mortality from pleurectomy/decortication is <2%, while mortality from extrapleural pneumonectomy has ranged from 6% to 30%.[2]

Radiation/Chemotherapy - The use of radiation therapy in pleural mesothelioma has been shown to alleviate pain in the majority of patients treated; however, the duration of symptom control is short-lived. Single-agent and combination chemotherapy have been evaluated in single and combined modality studies. The most studied agent is doxorubicin, which has produced partial responses in approximately 15% to 20% of patients studied. Some combination chemotherapy regimens have been reported to have higher response rates in small phase II trials; however, the toxic effects reported are also higher, and there is no evidence that combination regimens result in longer survival or longer control of symptoms.[3]

Alimta - The only FDA approved chemotherapy for malignant pleural mesothelioma (in combination with cisplatin) is pemetrexed (Alimta). In the key clinical trial that led to its approval, Alimta was combined with another chemotherapy drug (cisplatin) and compared with cisplatin alone. The median survival for the patients who received both drugs was 12.1 months versus 9.3 months for cisplatin only.[4]

Other Treatments – There are a number of FDA-approved clinical trials for the treatment of mesothelioma. For a list of trials currently recruiting patients see the National Cancer Institute website: http://www.cancer.gov/search/clinical_trials/

Sources:
Unless otherwise indicated by an endnote, the above medical material was adapted from National Cancer Institute Cancer Facts - Mesothelioma: Questions and Answers 5/13/2002.

Endnotes:
[1] National Cancer Institute Malignant Mesothelioma (PDQ®): Treatment; Health Professional Version
[2] Id.
[3] Id.
[4] Vogelzang NJ, et al., Phase III study of pemetrexed in combination with cisplatin versus cisplatin alone in patients with malignant pleural mesothelioma. J Clin Oncol. 2003 Jul 15;21(14):2636-44.

℘ Appendix Seven ℭ

MESOTHELIOMA AND THE IMMUNE SYSTEM

Paul Kraus is not the only long-term survivor of malignant mesothelioma. There are others. What is fascinating is that many long-term mesothelioma survivors appear to have something in common - they have taken steps to improve or enhance their immune system. For example, some patients used alternative or complementary therapies (with guidance from licensed clinicians) while others participated in clinical trials of immune therapies.

This raises the question - does the immune system play a role in controlling malignant mesothelioma? Paul Kraus' experience and those of some other long-term malignant mesothelioma survivors suggests that such a role may be possible.

In 1986, an article appeared in a medical journal that discussed this very issue.[1] The research focused on the immune responses of 118 healthy people compared to 20 patients with malignant mesothelioma and 375 long-term asbestos workers who were cancer-free. The researchers wanted to know if there were any measurable differences in the immune responses of the mesothelioma patients. Their findings suggested a relationship between the immune system and malignant mesothelioma. For example:

• The number of total T (T11+) and T-helper (T4+) cells were normal in asbestos workers without cancer, but were significantly reduced in patients with mesothelioma. T cells orchestrate, regulate and coordinate the overall immune response.

• Most patients with mesothelioma had a profound deficiency in Natural Killer cell (NK) activity which is suggestive of the role the immune system plays in the control of malignant mesothelioma. NK cells are a type of lethal lymphocyte that target tumor cells and protect against a wide variety of infectious microbes.

In the discussion section of the report, the researchers stated:

"These findings led us to speculate that biological phenomena generally categorized as chronic immunosuppression associated with the presence of asbestos fibers in the exposed workers may have caused the eventual breakdown of the host's surveillance system and the onset of neoplasm [malignant mesothelioma]."

The researchers are suggesting that malignant mesothelioma may ultimately result from immune suppression. If this is true it would provide the biological basis for the role that the immune system and immune boosting approaches may play in the management of malignant mesothelioma.

Case Histories of Long-Term Mesothelioma Survivors

Below are some case histories of cancer survivors who were diagnosed with either pleural or peritoneal mesothelioma. These case histories have been published in the peer reviewed medical literature and provide evidence that there are people that survive this disease for many years. In addition, in some of the pleural mesothelioma cases, doctors discuss the role that the patient's immune system may have played in their extremely long survival.

Pleural Mesothelioma

12 Years +

In 1994, a 58 year old man complained of chest pain and shortness of breath.[2] He had been exposed to asbestos

163

previously through his work and was eventually diagnosed with malignant pleural mesothelioma. The patient decided not to have any active treatment at that time and continued with his life. Five years later he had an enlarging painless mass on his chest wall. A needle biopsy confirmed it was malignant. The patient had a left thoracotomy, multiple pleural biopsies, and chest wall resection. Pathology reconfirmed that the mass was malignant pleural mesothelioma. Seven years after the chest wall resection and 12 years after the initial diagnosis, the patient has no symptoms and no evidence of recurrence. No chemotherapy or radiation had been given.

The doctors who wrote up this case history for publication noted that there was "moderate host inflammatory response" and that "spontaneous regression may be an immune-mediated phenomenon." The doctors hypothesized that the patient's own immune system may have played a role in his survival.

14 Years

In 1986, a 65 year-old women had pain in her left chest wall.[3] A chest X-ray revealed a small pleural effusion on this side. The patient declined an open biopsy and no diagnosis could be reached. She was treated for tuberculosis because of the high rate of this disease in her area. Her symptoms partially improved. In 1988 she had increasing pain over her chest. A biopsy was performed and malignant infiltration of the pleura was confirmed. She turned down treatment. In 1998, ten years after the diagnosis of malignant pleural mesothelioma she had an enlarging mass over her left chest wall. Biopsy confirmed the diagnosis of pleural mesothelioma. She had a course of radiation and died in January 2000, 14 years after her initial symptoms.

The doctors who wrote this report counseled their colleagues that long-term survivors can occur with pleural mesothelioma and "one should not hold the belief that it is always the intervention that prolongs survival." These doctors suggested that in some cases the intervention (i.e. chemotherapy, radiation, surgery) may not be the factor that prolongs survival in pleural mesothelioma, but other factors may be at work.

7 Years +

In 1970, a 53 year-old man had shortness of breath and a sharp pain on his right side.[4] An X-ray revealed a right side pleural effusion. The patient had worked at a plant adjacent to the Brooklyn Navy Yard from 1955-1966 where asbestos had been used. In 1972, a thoracotomy was performed and a pleural biopsy was taken. The patient was diagnosed with malignant pleural mesothelioma. The patient never received any specific treatment for pleural mesothelioma. The report was written up in 1977 and apparently information about the continued life of this patient was not published after that. We do not know how many more years or decades he lived.

The doctors noted in their discussion of this patient, "This unusual course may be explained either by the presence of low-grade malignancy or by the unusual host resistance…Our findings are consistent with the concept that normal immunological function may effectively impede dissemination of the disease (malignant pleural mesothelioma)." These doctors are again alluding to how the immune system may play a role in managing this cancer in some patients.

Peritoneal Mesothelioma

9 Years +

In November 1979, a 73 year-old man had abdominal pain and distension and was found to have an abdominal mass.[5] A laparotomy was performed that revealed peritoneal malignancy with ascites. A biopsy demonstrated that the tumor was malignant peritoneal mesothelioma. No special treatment was recommended other than draining of the ascites. In spite of the continuing ascites and the gradually-enlarging abdominal masses, the patient enjoys good health, and lives independently at home. How many more years (in excess of nine when this report was published) this patient lived is not known.

15 Years +

A woman was diagnosed with peritoneal mesothelioma. She had surgery ("total excision").[6] Seven years later the peritoneal mesothelioma recurred and she had another surgery ("reexcision"). She remains well 15 years after the initial diagnosis. The patient did not receive chemotherapy.

17 + Years

In 1962, a 31 year-old woman had abdominal pain for several months and a mass was detected.[7] She underwent exploratory laparotomy which found tumor nodules spread throughout her abdomen. The diagnosis of peritoneal mesothelioma was made. Complete surgical removal of the tumor was not possible. She was treated with radioactive phosphorus, radiation, and oral chemotherapy (cytoxan). She remained well for 17 years. In 1979 she had recurrent peritoneal mesothelioma. She was treated with cytoxan again and continued to live as of the writing of the published medical report.

The message from these case studies is clear – some patients do survive mesothelioma using a variety of approaches and therapies. In addition, in some patients, the response of their immune system may have been of importance.

Endnotes:
[1] Lew, F., et al., High Frequency of Immune Dysfunctions in Asbestos Workers and in Patients with Malignant Mesothelioma, Journal of Clinical Immunology; 1986, 6:3, 225-232.
[2] Pilling, J.E., et al., Prolonged Survival Due to Spontaneous Regression and Surgical Excision of Malignant Mesothelioma, Ann Thorac Surg, 2007; 83: 314-5.

[3] Wong, C.F., et al., A Case of Malignant Pleural Mesothelioma with Unexpectantly Long Survival without Active Treatment, Respiration March/April 2002; 69, 2: 166-168.

[4] Fischbein, A,. et al., Unexpected Longevity of a Patient with malignant Pleural Mesothelioma, Cancer 1978; 42:1999-2004.

[5] Norman, P.E. and Whitaker, D., Nine-Year Survival in a Case of Untreated Peritoneal Mesothelioma, Med J Aust 1989; 150: 43-44.

[6] Asensio, J.A., et al., Primary Malignant Peritoneal Mesothelioma: A Report of Seven Cases and a Review of the Literature, Arch Surg; Nov 1990, 125, 1477-1480.

[7] Brenner, J., et al., Seventeen Year Survival in a Patient with malignant Peritoneal Mesothelioma; Clinical Oncology 1981, 7, 249-251.

℘ Appendix Eight ℃

MESOTHELIOMA COMPENSATION

We are often asked questions about how mesothelioma compensation works. Below are some answers to frequently asked questions. If you would like tips on how to identify and interview reputable mesothelioma lawyers in your region, you may call the Client Services Team at MRHFM at 800-259-9249 and they can provide you with further information.

What is asbestos?

Asbestos is a naturally occurring mineral. It is resistant to heat and corrosion and it is made of fibers so it can be woven into other materials. American companies called it the "magic mineral" because it had so many uses. The other reason it is unique is because it is a carcinogen and it causes mesothelioma. When asbestos fibers get into the air they are invisible to the naked eye and can be easily inhaled or ingested. This may cause an asbestos related disease like mesothelioma years later.

Was asbestos used in the construction of homes and buildings?

Yes. Because of its resistance to heat and corrosion and the fact that it could be weaved and combined with other materials, asbestos was used in many different types of building materials. Paint, joint compound, insulation, flooring, roofing tiles, shingles, putty, even the reflectors around lights may have contained asbestos at one time. If your house or office was built before the mid 1970's it may still contain some asbestos containing products.

Where was asbestos used in the home?

In addition, to being in the construction materials used to build houses, buildings and other structures, asbestos was used in hundreds of different products used in the typical home. Baby bottle warmers, dish towels, oven mitts, hair dryers, stove liners, ironing boards and even children's cake-making sets contained asbestos in the past. Although most of these products no longer contain asbestos they were a familiar sight in the 1950's and 1960's.

Was asbestos ever used in cigarettes?

Yes, asbestos was used in at least one brand of cigarettes in the 1950's.

Can I get exposed to asbestos fibers from somebody else?

Yes, this is called secondary exposure. One example is the wife who washes her husband's dirty work clothes that are covered with invisible asbestos fibers. As she handles the clothes she may inhale or ingest some of the airborne fibers. There have been thousands of cases like this. Another example is the so-called "deadly hug." This happens when a child hugs their parent when he or she returns home from work and some asbestos is transferred to the child from the adult's work clothes. Unfortunately, there have been many cases like this as well.

Can I receive compensation even if I don't know how I was exposed to asbestos?

Many people do not know exactly how they were exposed to asbestos. After all, mesothelioma is usually diagnosed decades after the person came into contact with asbestos. Based on your work and residential history, reputable mesothelioma lawyers can help you piece it together. There have been approximately 40,000 cases of mesothelioma diagnosed in the U.S. in the last 20 years. This has led to the accumulation of vast amounts of knowledge about how people were exposed to asbestos in different towns, cities, states, occupations, and companies.

Why is there money available to mesothelioma victims?

Money is available because asbestos is considered the only cause of mesothelioma and it was put deliberately into products by companies that knew it was dangerous. Now, these companies have been caught and must pay for their decisions that killed and injured innocent victims. This is how our system of justice works. There is money potentially available from trust funds that were set-up by bankrupt companies and also from non-bankrupt companies.

Will I have to go to court?

There is the possibility of going to court, but it is statistically unlikely. The overwhelming majority of mesothelioma cases settle out of court. The decision as to whether to go to court is always the client's, the lawyer can only make a recommendation.

Is there any reason to file my claim or lawsuit right away?

Yes, the value of your case depends on the evidence. Where you worked or lived. What you did. What products you may have purchased or used. The best source of this evidence is the mesothelioma victim. It is advantageous to provide this information early in the diagnosis before the patient starts cancer treatment. In addition, there are statutes of limitations so you only have a limited amount of time to file your case or claim and the clock usually starts to tick on the day of diagnosis.

The entire subject of compensation can be overwhelming especially when the patient and their family are dealing with the stress of a recent diagnosis. However, picking the right attorney and protecting your legal rights can be very important. For example, receiving funds quickly can help a family pay for treatments not covered by insurance, lost wages, transportation, and to protect your family's financial security. The Client Services Team at MRHFM would be happy to walk you through the process and answer any questions you may have. You can reach them at 800-259-9249.

Mesothelioma By The Numbers:

- Approximately 3,000 mesothelioma cases a year.

- Over 40 trust funds set-up for asbestos and mesothelioma victims with approximately $30 billion available to patients.

- Estimated that $10 billion in total has already been paid out to thousands of asbestos victims.

❧ Appendix Nine ☙

USEFUL CONTACTS
AND RESOURCES

Cancer Monthly

Cancer Monthly provides cancer patients with the results of hundreds of therapies for advanced and metastatic cancers so that patients can compare treatments, have more meaningful discussions with their doctors, and ultimately, make more informed treatment decisions.

http://www.cancermonthly.com

National Cancer Institute

The National Cancer Institute coordinates the National Cancer Program, which conducts and supports research, training, health information dissemination, and other programs with respect to the cause, diagnosis, prevention, and treatment of cancer.

Cancer Overviews http://www.cancer.gov/cancertopics

Clinical Trials http://www.cancer.gov/clinicaltrials

Pubmed

PubMed is a service of the National Library of Medicine that includes over 15 million citations from MEDLINE and other life science journals for biomedical articles. PubMed includes links to full text articles and other related resources.

http://www.ncbi.nlm.nih.gov/entrez/query.fcgi

Surviving Mesothelioma
This website provides information on conventional therapies, biological therapies, immunotherapies, alternative treatments and clinics.
http://www.survivingmesothelioma.com

❧ Appendix Ten ❧

GLOSSARY

ACUPUNCTURE: Is routinely practiced in traditional Chinese medicine. It consists of placing needles at key points – 'energy meridians' along the body in order to restore the vital balance between the ying and the yang energy levels. Acupuncture is commonly used in pain control and to alleviate the symptoms of many other conditions, including sinusitis and gynecological problems.

ADENOCARCINOMA: A carcinoma of glandular origin. (Refer also to 'carcinoma.')

ADJUNCTIVE THERAPIES: Therapies that complement conventional or orthodox cancer treatments.

ASCITES: Accumulation of fluid in the abdominal cavity.

BIOFEEDBACK: A technique used by certain health professionals, including doctors, that 'feeds back' to us information showing what goes on in our bodies when we think or feel certain things.

CARCINOMA: A malignant tumor originating in the tissues that line the organs of the body such as the pancreas, kidneys, liver and skin.

COMPLEMENTARY THERAPIES: Those forms of therapy that fall outside the conventional forms of cancer treatment. Some of these, such as nutritional therapy stand alongside traditional therapies such as chemotherapy or radiation treatment.

CONVENTIONAL CANCER THERAPY: Traditionally, these forms of therapy include surgery, chemotherapy and radiation.

DETOXIFICATION: Variety of practices designed to rid the body of accumulated toxins. For example, juicing, eating fresh organic fruit and vegetables.

DYSPLASIA: Abnormal changes in cells.

EPITHELIUM: The tissue that lines the surfaces of the body's organs.

GERSON DIET: Nutritional treatment based on achieving a favorable sodium/potassium balance by restricting fat and protein consumption.

HODGKIN'S DISEASE: A malignant condition of the lymph tissues that results in the enlargement of the lymph nodes, spleen and liver.

IMAGERY: The use of mental images that come to conscious awareness during a deeply relaxed state to motivate the body's healing response.

ISCADOR: A mistletoe extract, used widely in Europe, as an anti-cancer agent.

LYMPHOMA: A malignant growth originating in the lymph tissues.

MACROBIOTICS: A form of diet that is grain-based and nondairy, primarily cooked and usually vegetarian.

MELANOMA: A malignant form of skin cancer.

METABOLIC DISEASE: One in which the body fails to convert digested nutrients into energy or building blocks for tissue regeneration.

METASTASES: Locations where cancer has spread from its primary site, usually via the lymph system or blood.

MICRONUTRIENTS: Vitamins and trace minerals.

MYELOMA: A primary tumor originating in the bone marrow.

NEOPLASM: The word actually refers to a new growth.

PALLIATIVE: Treatment that provides relief from symptoms, as distinct from a cure.

PAVLOVIAN: Refers to the technique of conditioned reflexes, pioneered by Russian physiologist I P Pavlov.

REMISSION: The diminution, or lessening, of a disease such as cancer.

SARCOMA: Cancer of the connective tissues, including bone.

TRANS-FATTY ACIDS: Lipid (fat or oil) molecules that have been hydrogenated or heated to high temperatures (such as oil used for frying or the fat in margarine) are as harmful as saturated fats (bacon, cheese, steaks) because they stop cells functioning properly.

ℬ

BIBLIOGRAPHY

Cousins, N, *Anatomy of an Illness*, Bantam Books, New York, 1980.

Backus, William, *The Healing Power of a Christian Mind*, Bethany House, Minnesota, USA, 1996.

Borysenko, Joan and Boryenko, Miroslav, *The Power of the Mind to Heal*, Warner Books, New York, 1994.

Hirshberg, Caryle, and Barasch, Marc Ian, *Remarkable Recovery: What Extraordinary Healings Can Tell Us About Getting Well and Staying Well*, Hodder Headline, London, 1995.

Gawler, Ian, *You Can Conquer Cancer*, Hill of Content, Melbourne, 1984.

Gawler, Ian, *Peace of Mind*, Hill of Content, Melbourne, 1987.

Gawler, Ian, (ed.), *Inspiring People*, Hill of Content, Melbourne, 1995.

Horne, Ross, *Cancerproof Your Body*, Allen & Unwin, Sydney, 1989.

King, Petrea, *Quest for Life*, Random House, Sydney, 1988.

Kraus, Paul, *Faith, Hope, Love and Laughter – How They Heal*, Hale & Iremonger, Sydney, 1999.

Lerner, Michael, *Choices in Healing: Integrating the Best of Conventional and Complementary Approaches to Cancer*, MIT Press, Cambridge, Massachusetts, 1996.

Nathan, Joel, *What to do when they say 'It's cancer.': A Survivor's Guide*, Allen & Unwin, Sydney, 1998.

Meares, A., *Cancer, Another Way?*, Hill of Content, Melbourne, 1977.

MacNutt, Francis, *Healing*, Creation House Publishing, Jacksonville, Florida, 1988.

Pert, Candace, *Molecules of Emotion: The Science Behind Mind–Body Medicine*, Touchstone Books, Simon & Schuster, New York, 1999.

Siegel, Bernie, *Peace, Love and Healing*, Arrow Books, London, 1991.

Siegel, Bernie, *Love, Medicine and Miracles*, Arrow Books, London, 1988.

Simonton, Carl, and Matthews-Simonton, Stephanie, *Getting Well Again*, Bantam Books, New York, 1992.

ॐ

PERMISSIONS

Extract from *Love, Medicine and Miracles* by Bernie Siegel, published by Century. Used with the permission of The Random House Group Limited.

Extract from *Prescriptions for Living* by Bernie Siegel published by HarperCollins. Used with permission.

Extracts from *You Can Conquer Cancer* by Ian Gawler, published by Hill of Content. Used with permission.

Extracts from *Choices in Healing* by Michael Lerner, published by MIT Press. Used with permission.
Extract from *Getting Well Again*, by Carl and Stephanie Simons, published by Bantam Books.

Extract from *Spontaneous Healing* by Andrew Weil, published by Random House. Used with permission.

Brief extracts from *Molecules of Emotion*, by Candace Pert, published by Simon and Schuster, New York.

Brief extract from *Quest for Life* by Petrea King, published by Random House.

Every effort has been made to contact copyright holders. The publisher would be pleased to hear from any copyright holder where unintentional infringement has occurred due to difficulty in tracing the copyright holder.

ℬ

INDEX

consciousness, 55, 58, 99,
    100, 107
conventional therapies,
    20
    limitations, 65
Dean Ornish, 48
decortication, 160
detoxification, 84, 85, 91
diagnosis, 12, 68
    accepting, 14
    initial response, 98
Diagnosis, 159
diet, 21, 84
    changes, 67
    choices, 82
    digestion, 85
    fats, 87
    flaxseed oil, 93
    healing, 83, 86
    individual, 84
    maintenance, 84
    organic, 86
    protein, 88
    vegetarian, 89
doctor
    selection, 67
doctor patient
    relationship, 21
eating
    choices, 62
efficacy, 20
emotions
    acknowledging, 60
    definitions, 58

digestion, 62
    healing, 59
employment, 11
enzymes, 90, 91, 95
exercises, 33, 34, 43, 44,
    46, 59, 61, 64, 76, 102,
    103, 105, 106, 108, 117
Extrapleural
    Pneumonectomy, 16,
    160
faith, 29
    paradox, 59
    trust, 29
faith factor'
    recoveries, 30
fear, 13
Flaxseed Oil, 95
forgiveness, 11, 30, 32,
    41, 42, 43, 44, 61, 64,
    112, 118
Gawler Foundation, 39,
    126
German medical model,
    69
Gerson Diet, 82, 84
Gerson Therapy, 91
ginseng tea, 78
gratitude, 45
green tea, 78
gut feeling, 57
healer, 22
herbal
    medicine, 76, 77
    supplement, 92